What early readers said about this book.

Refusing to be defined by cancer, Professor Roberts challenges readers to reframe our thinking about the disease and how we respond to it. This collection of essays is written with sensitivity, intellectual acuity, and profound authenticity. It is a must read for all who are affected by cancer: patient, family, friends, medical, and pastoral practitioners. -Dr. Robert G. Rogers, Professor Emeritus of Religion and Lay Pastoral Care Associate.

* * * * * * *

This is a remarkable book of great generosity and honesty and hope, written for you, for me, for our loved ones when serious disease enters our lives. Roberts chooses his own path to healing, including the modern medicine of the Mayo Clinic, meditation, diet, qigong treatments, prayer. He chooses his own language and metaphors, forgoing the militaristic words often employed when dealing with cancer. He chooses to continue his teaching and his political action work, using every ounce of energy allotted each day. He chooses community, not isolation; humor, not dread. He chooses how to understand God's powerful presence in this struggle. Roberts' intensity never falters: Life is too rich in meaning and purpose.-Sarah Campbell Lead Minister, Mayflower UCC Church, Minneapolis

* * * * * * *

Keith Roberts shares his analysis as a sociologist and his innermost feelings as a human being as he processes what it means to have stage IV cancer. The result is a thought-provoking read for any person contemplating the meaning of suffering and illness. He encourages all of us to "make meaning" of whatever life throws at us. *Maggie Cupit, author Why God? Suffering through Cancer into Fai...

* * * * * * *

Traversing the paths of physical treatments and mental states, anyone involved in "making meaning" of illness will find this book thoughtful, realistic, and inspiring. Medical, religious, and other support groups, as well as individuals facing life challenges will find this book thought-provoking and a chance to delve into issues related to their new status, or that of a friend or loved one. Like ruminations by another sociologist (*Tuesdays with Morrie*) regarding life's struggles, Keith Roberts takes us on a journey that explores philosophical, theological, psychological, and sociological aspects of living meaningfully. *-Jeanne Ballantine, Sociology Professor Emerita, Wright State University*

* * * * * * *

Keith Roberts has given us an extraordinary book about his journey with cancer and meaning making. Persons of different religious backgrounds will gain many insights and benefits from his philosophical and theological perspectives on a challenging and spiritual journey. *-Dr. Robert E. Reber, former Dean and professor at Auburn Theological Seminary in New York City, and founder of the Center for Multifaith Education.*

* * * * * * *

Keith Roberts' *Meaning Making with Malignancy* is a life-enriching book on death and suffering. With thought-provoking sociological and theoretical reflections, interwoven with Roberts's personal experience with cancer, it helps us to make sense of not just an advanced cancer diagnosis, but our very lives. In doing so, it provides comfort and meaning during challenging and life-threatening times. *Meaning Making with Malignancy* is for cancer patients, caretakers, sociologists, theologians, and anyone looking for inspiration. *-Dr. Kathleen Odell Korgen, Professor of Sociology, William Patterson University.*

* * * * * * *

MEANING-MAKING WITH MALIGNANCY

A Theologically Trained Sociologist Reflects
on Living Meaningfully with Cancer

KEITH A. ROBERTS

ISBN 978-1-64003-748-9 (Paperback)
ISBN 978-1-64003-749-6 (Digital)

Covenant Books, Inc.
11661 Hwy 707
Murrells Inlet, SC 29576
www.covenantbooks.com

Special permissions for quotes or use of images granted from:

Margaret Carlisle Cupit, Edward Henderson, and David Hein, *Why, God? Suffering Through Cancer into Faith*. Eugene, OR: Wipf and Stock Publishers, 2015, [94-95]. ISBN 978-162564-478-7 www.wip-fandstock.com; Robin Wall Kimmerer's *Braiding Sweetgrass: Indigenous Wisdom, Scientific Knowledge, and the Teachings of Plants*. Minneapolis, MN: Milkweed Editions. Copyright 2013 by Robin Kimmerer. Reprinted with permission from Milkweed Editions. milkweed.org; Howard Thurman. "For a Time of Sorrow" pp. 211-212 in *Meditations of the Heart*. Boston: Beacon Press. Copyright 1953, 1981 by Anne Thurman. Reprinted by permission of Beacon Press, Boston; and CartoonStock and John **Deering** for use of cartoons in chapter 15.

CONTENTS

Introduction...9

1. Health Crisis—Positive Energies Needed 13
2. Who Have I Not Told? 17
3. Allopathy and Alternative Approaches to Healing 21
4. Framing One's Reality and Plausibility Structures 26
5. Why Me? Why Us? Micro and Macro Malignancies 41
6. Faith, Values, and Healing 48
7. Paradigms and Constructions of Reality..............................54
8. Living with Ambiguity...59
9. How Do I Name This Experience? Warlike and
   Non-warlike Metaphors 66
10. Awkward!—What to Say
    (or Not Say) to Friends with a Life-threatening Disease 74
11. The Challenge of Cancer to a Coherent and Healthy Self........86
12. Planning for the Future When "Planning the Future"
    Feels like an Oxymoron 95
13. Communicating and Living One's Legacy............................104
14. Optimism or Hope? Some Dilemmas and Ironies 114
15. Levity, Laughter, Humor (including Tumor Humor).............121
16. Hope and Healing: Omnipotence? Really? 133
17. Meaning Matters..142

References 149
Appendix: Questions for a Cancer Support Group 153

INTRODUCTION

Three days before Thanksgiving, 2016, I sent off the final manuscript for a coauthored sixth edition of an introduction to sociology textbook, *Our Social World*. Two days later—the day before Thanksgiving—I went in for a routine procedure to expand or "dilate" my esophagus, a procedure my mother, our oldest son, and my siblings had undergone to correct problems related to swallowing. Instead, the gastroenterologist discovered a "black fuzzy mass" that he was pretty sure was malignant. He took a biopsy, and I went immediately for a CT scan. The day after Thanksgiving, I received the news that not only was the mass malignant but that it had spread to my lungs and lymph nodes. I, who had always been as healthy as a horse, had stage 4 cancer.

The first few weeks—even the first month—was a foggy blur of trying to figure out which oncologist, which cancer center, what forms of alternative or integrative medicine, and other decisions were navigated. In less than two weeks, I was scheduled for my first chemotherapy treatments at the Mayo Clinic in Rochester, Minnesota, just ninety minutes from our home. I would be in a recliner with intravenous tubes pumping poison into my system for four hours every other week. I decided to take my laptop and use that time writing to family and friends about my situation. Very quickly, I found that summarizing my medical update was not enough; in fact, I found it quite boring. I was filled with questions about what all of this means. How do I make sense of what I have been experiencing? So each entry began with brief updates on my own health and health care; I followed it with reflections or musings on what all of this meant. Initially, I called this "Keith's Kancer Chronicles." I started by mailing these to perhaps two dozen family and friends, but I found they forwarded my musings to others, and I was quickly expanding the e-mailing list to several hundred. I was even informed that an oncology nurse in Hawaii was distributing these musings to her cancer patients.

As a sociologist—one who also has an advanced degree in theology—I found that constructing meaning came rather naturally. Humans need meaning to make sense of their lives, and this is especially true as we find ourselves in highly ambiguous or threatening situations. The essays that follow are what I sent to family and friends as I moved though this engagement with cancer. My readers strongly encouraged me to find a publisher. This book is the result. As these reflections began to look like they might become a book, I decided to keep the personal medical updates since those ground the essays in specific time and events that gave rise to many of the ruminations.

In *Braiding Sweetgrass: Indigenous Wisdom, Scientific Knowledge, and the Teachings of Plants*, Robin Wall Kimmerer discusses returning to her Potawatomi people after completing a Ph.D. in botany and she contrasts some of the meanings imbedded in languages, in his case English and Potawatomi (which is closely related to Ojibwe).

Kimmerer's native language forces the speaker to distinguish inanimate objects (expressed as nouns) from animate subjects (expressed as verbs). Moreover, there are not many noun forms in Ojibwa, but there are *many* verbs.

> [In] the Ojibwa dictionary… all kinds of things seemed to be verbs: "to be a hill," "to be red," "to be a long sandy stretch of beach," and then my finger rested on *wiikwegamaa*: "to be a bay." Ridiculous!" I ranted in my head. "There is no reason to make it so complicated… A bay is most definitely a person, place, or thing—a noun and not a verb."
>
> And then I swear I heard a zap of synapses firing… A bay is a noun only if it is *dead*. When a *bay* is a noun, it is defied by humans, trapped between its shores and contained by the word. But the verb *wiikwegamaa*—to *be* a bay—releases the water from bondage and lets it live. "To be a bay holds

the wonder that, for this moment, the living water has decided to shelter itself between these shores... Water, land... the language [is] a mirror for seeing the animacy of the world, the life that pulses through all things, through pines and nuthatches and mushrooms.

This is the language of animacy. Imagine seeing your grandmother standing at the stove in her apron and then saying of her, "Look, it is making soup. It has gray hair." We might snicker at such a mistake, but we also recoil from it. In English, we never refer to a member of our family, or indeed to any person, as *it*. That would be a profound act of disrespect. It robs a person of selfhood and kinship, reducing a person to a mere thing... Doesn't this mean that speaking English, thinking in English, somehow gives us permission to disrespect nature? By denying everyone else the right to be [a subject]? Wouldn't things be different if nothing was an *it*?... If a maple is an *it*, we can take up the chain saw. If a maple is a *she*, we think twice.

(From *Braiding Sweetgrass* by Robin Wall Kimmerer (Minneapolis: Milkweed Editions, 2013), pp. 54-57. Copyright © 2013 by Robin Wall Kimmerer. Reprinted with permission from Milkweed Editions. milkweed.org)

Kimmerer found that her native language compelled her to think differently about the natural world and humanity's relationship to it. In short, the language created different meaning. When we rethink what things mean—how we define *reality*—it may prod us to change how we respond to our life circumstances. Is stage 4 cancer the same thing as terminal cancer? If so, how do we respond? If not, what difference might that make in how we approach treatment? These are the kinds of reflections I undertake in these musings.

KEITH A. ROBERTS

In some of the following chapters, I focus on advice to people who have a chronically ill friend or family member. An example is the chapter, "Awkward! What to Say (or Not Say) to Friends with a Life-threatening Disease." On other occasions, I reflect on the experience of having a life-threatening disease, and my audience is others in that situation. Examples of chapters with this focus would include "Planning for the Future When 'Planning the Future' Feels like an Oxymoron," "Living with Ambiguity," and "How Do I Name This Experience? Warlike and Non-warlike Metaphors." The reflections are sometimes informed by philosophical or theological analyses but more often by a sociological lens.

I found this writing itself to be somewhat therapeutic for me, but the depth and breadth of the response from readers made me think that others might find these ruminations useful. The chaplains and counselors at the Mayo Clinic indicated that they have very little that they can recommend to people with cancer for reading or for use in a cancer support group. The back of this book includes "starter" questions that a support group might find useful in discussing their own struggles.

I do hope that you find this insightful as you try to cope and find meaning in the abyss of a chronic illness like cancer.

Keith A. Roberts
Emeritus Professor of Sociology and Anthropology
Hanover College

1

Health Crisis—Positive Energies Needed

December 9, 2016

Hi, family and dear friends.

Judy and I have been so appreciative of the phenomenal support we have received as we have experienced this unexpected encounter with cancer. There are so very many people who have written that I am sending this out as a general update, but I certainly do not want to overwhelm people with updates or information. If you would like to be updated in the future, let us know, and we will add you to the list. Otherwise, this will serve as the report on my status.

Since some of you have had quite recent updates and others have heard little, I will risk some redundancy. Two weeks ago, a procedure to remove acid reflux scar tissue from my esophagus (so I could swallow) discovered instead a malignant esophageal tumor. The CT scan showed the cancer was also in my lung and lymph glands, so it is systemic. Since I have had truly extraordinary health all my life (missing only one class in forty years of college teaching), it has been a shock and has turned our lives upside down. One quickly starts to assess priorities.

We have consulted doctors at three major and nationally respected cancer centers, have discussed diet with a naturopathic physician, have people doing Reiki for me, have had a two-hour session with a Qigong master (a four-thousand -year-old traditional Chinese medicine practice that focuses on exercises with meditation, massage, and diet to influence energy flow in the body), and have employed energy healing practices that are in line with insights from quantum physics. So we are addressing this from multiple angles. The conventional "allopathy" doctors call this a "stage 4" cancer, and the focus is on palliative rather than curative care. Still, there is about a 1 percent chance of cure, and given all the support I have and my excellent health in all other respects, I am expecting to be in a best-case scenario (even while we change our life priorities).

The support we have received, especially through the Mayflower Church in Minneapolis and also from *so many other* people whose lives we have crossed, is phenomenal. The support has been very heartening and encouraging. Thank you, thank you, and thank you!

I write this from the Mayo Clinic hooked up to a chemo intravenous machine, wrapped in the warm (in more ways than one) crocheted prayer shawl given to us from our church community. It is large enough that Judy and I (sometimes our son from Anchorage too) can be wrapped in it for a morning meditation period each day. After consulting three very excellent cancer centers, we have decided to, at least, begin with Dr. Pitot and his colleagues at the Mayo Clinic. Mayo is ranked the number 1 hospital in North America and third in the country for cancer treatment. It is truly a very impressive international medical center and has more likelihood of having clinical trials with new drugs and treatments than most places. Mayo is ninety minutes from our home, but a number of people have already offered to drive me so the transport does not all fall on Judy. Borrowing a term from dear friend Carla Howery, I call these chemo friends my chemo-sabes (remember the Lone Ranger and Tonto?).

My initial regimen is a two-week cycle with intravenous chemo every other week followed by carrying a pump with me that infuses another drug for forty-six hours. Then I have twelve days with nothing. I am told it is highly unlikely that I will experience nausea, or even hair loss, with the chemical combination and with the newer anti-nausea meds. I will probably continue with Qigong treatment, daily meditation, and close attention to diet.

Niece Bethan and Mayflower friends Dr. Bob Scott and biologist Jeff Hughes had given me a valuable heads-up to ask about genetic coding work (in some places called precision medicine), which does DNA work and then matches chemical treatments to targeted indicators of the DNA. It is a very hopeful new area of cancer treatment, but, at least, at the Mayo, they view cancer as frequently a complex mixture of genetic and environmental factors with only about 15 percent of all cancers being solely rooted in biology. They will do the DNA work at stage 2 of treatment but felt that with an aggressive cancer such as I have, they should get started with killing cancer and shrinking the tumor. The good news is that they have already identified an extremely important DNA marker. I have HER2, which is a genetic cancer-prone factor, and this knowledge is very important for knowing how to attack cancer at the biological/genetic level. Mayo seems well positioned to treat this cancer from so many angles. We are blessed to be living in Minnesota where the medical community is so remarkably strong.

Other than an emotional roller coaster and some difficulty swallowing, I feel *great*. I feel as if Judy and I could again hike the forty-six kilometers Inca trail to Machu Picchu! We do still plan a trip to Costa Rica in January, so there is much positive future orientation deep in our souls. Although I have my moments, I am trying to sustain a positive, forward-looking attitude. I am planning to switch most of my writing efforts in a more personal direction—letters to grandkids, etc. that I should have been doing anyway—rather than so much focus on revising and publishing college textbooks.

All of this, or course, has been a deep shock to Judy and creates an unexpected life pivot for her. In some ways, I think we have each been more concerned about the impact of this diagnosis on the other than we have been on ourselves, so your prayers and various forms of support for her are *greatly* appreciated by me. She has such a generous heart that I am concerned that she take care of herself too. Our son, Justin, came from Alaska as soon as he heard about the diagnosis, and he will be with us for a month. Daughter Elise, Brett, and two-and-a-half-year-old Ramona live just ten minutes away from us, and that is huge. Each of them is enormously supportive. Justin's wife and fifteen-month old daughter Adina are also with us right now—a wonderful distraction. Second son Kent will arrive from Texas, along with Amanda and grandson Zain in a couple of weeks. Kent is actually thinking he may well move to Minneapolis to be nearby and provide additional support.

I deeply appreciate the many cards, letters, calls, e-mails, meals, gifts, and offers of help that have been coming in. We also received a wonderful knot blanket from our Huron Indiana Methodist community. This week has been a whirlwind during which decisions had to be made, and I could not respond to so many of the notes, but do know that you are appreciated!

This is a long missal—too long for most of you. I will not bother you with further updates unless I hear that you *specifically request* to be on an update list. Then we will try to be judicious in sending key updates. Please join me in trying to focus on the positive. Positive energy with imagining of healthiness enhances healing. Two days ago, I nearly fell into a solo "pity party" for myself (we were at the Mayo working through the system), and I saw two young people—probably twentyish—who were obviously *very* ill with cancer. It was sobering and made me appreciate my longevity and health to date. Judy and I have also been on human rights delegations to Global South countries like Honduras, Guatemala, and Colombia, and we know what both real suffering and profound resilience look like. My life has been and continues to be *very rich and full* I can only be grateful for the good fortune/privilege in my life and move forward with positive energy and hope for the future. Thanks for being part of this abundant path Judy and I have been on.

Peace and love,
Keith (and Judy) Roberts

2

Who Have I Not Told?

December 23, 2016

Family, friends,

Thanks to all the folks who have been so very responsive to Judy, to me, and to our kids as we face this cancer challenge. We are in good spirits (well, most of the time). This note is intended as an update, including how we are coping emotionally and how we seek to make sense of things.

I am again in the infusion room getting my second intravenous chemo treatment. In some ways, it has been a tough two weeks. Over about three months, I have lost twenty pounds—half of that has been since the last infusion, two weeks ago. I was extremely ill a week ago. We think that was a flu bug since two days after my first infusion, I was the only "healthy" person in the household. I cared for our fifteen-month-old granddaughter while Justin, Miriam, and Judy were down and out. I was hit five days later. I have gained seven of the ten pounds back, and I am probably only five pounds below what should be an ideal weight for me in the first place, so let's just say I am down about five pounds. I had five days when I could not eat much of anything, but my nutrition and energies are both "surging." (For those offering prayers and "imaging," my main problem right now is having very low white blood cells. I need to grow 'em!)

* * * * * *

In terms of coping and making sense of our situation, I think I should say first something about my diagnosis: stage 4 esophageal cancer. Until I had cancer myself, I think I tended to hear "stage 4 cancer" as a synonym for "terminal cancer." However, I would like to offer a more nuanced way to view my situation. Stage 4 includes people in a fairly wide set of circumstances: those who have massive systemic cancer in many organs, lymph nodes, and bloodstream and those who have cancer in two contiguous organs, which means the cancer is metastasized but not spread very far. My cancer is in my esophagus, lungs, and no doubt the lymph nodes, so the situation is serious, but I think it is premature to call it *terminal* cancer. That gives it too much power! I have too much yet to do—including justice work Judy and I are engaged in and some personal writing I intend to do. The term "terminal cancer" sounds like one already has one foot out the door. I don't! I am fully engaged and just this week testified at a hearing on racism in the criminal justice sentencing system... Well, a friend (Gini Johnson) actually read the testimony for me, but I wrote it and may need to deliver it myself at a subsequent legislative hearing in 2017. In short, I am vibrant and alive and moving forward. So please do not think of me in morbid terms or hold an image of me as "terminally ill." I may be *interminably* optimistic and long-winded in these missals, but I like to think that is different from being *terminal*. I will not be defined by the latter.

I am receiving Qigong treatments (Chinese exercise/movement, massage of acupressure points on the body, and meditation), mediating daily, making dramatic changes to an anticancer diet, receiving *energy healing* treatments (including but not limited to Reiki), reading extensively on cancer and how to either defeat or arrest it, and (per *prescription* of both our sons) watching lots of comedy. (Remember Norman Cousins laughing himself into good health?) Now, some of the research on diet and such do not satisfy the high standards of allopathic medicine evidence, but the instances of cures are also beyond just a few anecdotes with some statistical indications that show recovery is not totally out of reach using dietary changes. I highly recommend a book that a college friend, Joel Wingard, put me onto by the Director of the Center for Integrative Medicine at University of Pittsburgh, *Anticancer: A New Way of Life* (David Servan-Schreiber; Viking Press). I know you will be deeply sympathetic with the idea of drastic change in eating habits, but one of the painful realities is that among the best things for cancer is dark chocolate (over 70 percent cocoa). Tough sledding, but *someone* has to help keep the fair trade chocolate industry thriving! I have volunteered.

Most of us believe in the placebo effect. People sometimes recover when given a placebo simply because they expect to. My sister, Joyce, likes to point out the predictions of "how long one has to live" are often pretty accurate, and this may well be because of a *reverse placebo effect.* If one thinks one is dying, if one thinks she only has two months to live, why is this not like the placebo effect? We too often live out the expectation. So, folks, I do not have "terminal cancer"; I have stage 4 cancer, and I am working hard to either reverse or eliminate that from my "resume." My mother had a hot pot trivet in her kitchen that said, "Laughter is good medicine." Help me laugh about this cancer; it's good medicine for all of us.

David Servan-Schreiber reports on some empirical studies that are pretty strong evidence that positive attitudes have a powerful effect on retarding cancer and prolonging life, not to mention the way it buoys one's *quality* of life. The most important attitudinal factor is *agency* (the capacity to act or exert power as opposed to despair and sense of hopelessness). I wish you all a strong sense of *agency* for the coming year; we will surely need it as palpable incarnated evil takes over our government and must be resisted.

Finally, I have been getting some truly remarkable notes from people. Some have not just surprised me, they have shocked me. Some folks—including admired colleagues—have written to me about ways that I have affected their lives. Sometimes I find myself being floored, flabbergasted, and/or dumbfounded. It is very nice and very sweet and does much for a merry heart (also good medicine). I do not write this just to say how kind people have been with their words. Instead, I am struck with how seldom we tell people how much we admire them or how much they have been an unwitting model for us. As I read the kind words of others, I kept thinking, *Who have I not told?* There are so very many people who have inspired me, tutored me, modeled integrity for me—including most of the people on this mailing list. Often we wait until someone faces a life-threatening illness to tell him or her (or we wait until the funeral). But why?

Who have I not told? I am going to try to start whittling down that list. Although I may not get to each of you personally, you have meant and mean a great deal to me. Thank you for ways you have helped me to develop as a person (*and* as a professional).

Who have *you* not told? That might be a pretty extraordinary holiday gift—the gift of deep appreciation expressed to someone who has had a significant (perhaps transformative) influence on your life. Let's start giving that gift before that special someone has a life-threatening ailment!

Peace and love. Happy Solstice, Hanukah, Christmas, and (belatedly) *Milad un Nabi*. Eleven Robertses will gather here in Minneapolis and send you wishes for peace, justice, hope, and sustainability.

Keith

3

Allopathy and Alternative Approaches to Healing

January 6, 2017

Family, friends,

First, if anyone you know wants to be added to this list, let me know the e-mail address. Likewise, if anyone wants to be dropped, I will certainly take no offense, as we are all bombarded with more e-mail messages than we can process. Just drop me a line. You also all know where the delete button is!

I am again at the Mayo Clinic beginning another infusion. Two weeks ago, the doctor said one of my white blood cell indicators (neutrophils) was dangerously low. It was 1,080 (and should be over 1,500), and if that number did not improve, they would have to cancel my next chemo infusion. My family was plying me with all kinds of foods that build white blood cells, and many people have been offering prayers and sending energy my way. This week, that particular white blood cell indicator was over two thousand, and all other blood indicators where "high normal." While I have some nausea and low energy for a few days the week after infusion, the second week I feel fine—fit as a fiddle, so they say. We have radically changed my diet, I am getting acupressure massages and other forms of alternative healing, and our spirits overall are very good. We are resuming seminormal lives, and in a week and a half, I will be teaching a class on the Philosophy, Theology, and Ethics of Martin Luther King: the Role of Personalism in King's Thinking and the Civil Rights Movement. We are also taking several courses, such as one on film and spirituality. We are determined that cancer will not define our lives. We leave in just over two weeks for an ecotourism park in Costa Rica for five days to celebrate our seventieth birthdays. Life is good.

I might add that in the last week, I had a regular physical with my family doctor that included reports on a recent echocardiogram, a colonoscopy, and extensive blood tests. He said that if he did not have the oncology report right in front of him, he would say I was in excellent health, so I am perfectly positioned to beat the odds. As Stephen Jay Gould wrote on cancer diagnoses, "The median is not the message."

* * * * * * *

Some of you may only want to know *how* we are doing, and I report that at the outset of these chronicles, but to me, the more interesting issue is how one makes sense of all of this and forges ahead. So that is the second half of these chronicles from my perspective. If you are less interested in the musings of a nerdy professor, you may want to stop here.

Daughter Elise gave me a card that expresses one aspect of our "meaning-making." The card said, "Let me be the first to punch in the face the next person who says, 'Everything happens for a reason.'" While meant to be humorous, it does represent how we see this. The notion that "this is all part of God's plan" is deeply offensive—even blasphemous. That would be a very mean-spirited God, indeed. Not everything happens for a reason; life sometimes has randomness to it, and that means accidents and illnesses simply occur. While these events are not meaningful in themselves, meaning can be found and explored in any situation or circumstance, including realigning life priorities in a way that may be quite positive. Our task is to muddle through the circumstances we are experiencing, the conflicting information about treatments and strategies, and move forward with *agency* and *positive energy*.

Sometimes when I sit with Western or allopathic doctors, I feel like I am thrown back to debates I have had with professors with whom I have cotaught courses—especially psychologists—about how we know something (i.e. epistemology). Often they would deny that anything was known unless it was tested in an experimental laboratory (where variables could be controlled). They were often dismissive of other scientific (sociological) methods that study people who are "in the field" living their everyday lives. They would deny that observational studies of people, ethnographies, content analyses, and even statistical analyses of survey data were meaningful or scientific. They often seemed to me to be studying something they could control rather than something that mattered in people's lives. There are multiple ways and multiple strategies for understanding human life, each with special insights and each with blind spots. Laboratory studies also have blind spots, in part because people do not live their lives in controlled laboratories!

Likewise, allopathic Western doctors seem to think that nothing is established unless there have been multiple replications of studies with very large populations involving double blind crossover methodologies. They seem to dismiss everything else as "anecdotal." Allopathy has made *huge* contributions to our medical knowledge and health, but this is a huge blind spot in the allopathic view of reality. Moreover, their standard of "evidence" is so very restrictive that studies are dismissed if several variables are at work at once. It is not "objective" enough. One oncologist I talked to did not want me utilizing multiple methods (alternative approaches) because then we would not know *which one worked!* On the contrary, I like to see myself as a subject, not just an object in a set of controls. (My own oncologist is not so close-minded.) Frankly, when it comes to my health, I don't give a damn if every variable is controlled, and in fact, I suspect that the greatest health impacts are due to the synergy of several strategies that are used simultaneously. Indeed, Dr. Servan-Schreiber found that studies on the cumulative and synergistic effects of chemo, meditation, dietary changes, acupressure, regular exercise, and positive attitudes and sense of agency are much more effective than any one of these. Yet these studies are often dismissed in allopathic circles because they do not fit the very restrictive definitions of "evidence." It is as though many doctors have put on blinders, and they only study what they can measure with great precision. That is a problem. This is also a source of profound epistemological arrogance.

Judy and I are highly critical of many approaches, but we are convinced that double-blind crossover studies are not the only way to gain insight. We are convinced, for example, by rather highly sophisticated statistical analyses that meditation and positive attitudes have healing power. Indeed, high-tech research shows that when one controls one's breathing in meditation, the heartbeat and many other unconscious but necessary body processes begin to merge into a rhythmic symmetry, and this has profoundly positive health consequences (Servan-Schreiber, *Anticancer: A New Way of Life*, pp. 161–175).

Even if meditation and positive attitudes did not have healing power, they improve one's quality of life. In that spirit, let me share with you one of the Qigong exercises I most like. (Qigong is pronounced che-gong; the more widely known tai-chi is an offshoot of the more ancient Qigong.) One stands with hands folded as one might see Japanese men fold hands before bowing to one another. One then bends forward at the waist (as far or slight as is comfortable) and breathes in on the way down while thinking, *I am so grateful*. One exhales in the rising back to the upright position and mentions one thing that is a source of richness or blessing in one's life. One first goes through each of one's body parts and organs. (How often do we appreciate our *amazing* hearts or our feet or our digestive systems or our brains?) If quantum physics is correct that positive *thoughts* do affect objects in surprising ways, then directing appreciative thoughts to one's body can only be for the good. After appreciating one's body, one then goes through people, communities, events, relationships, and so forth that have added richness to one's life. The physical act of bowing keeps one's mind focused, and the overall impact is to create a deep sense of gratitude for all that is good in one's life. It generates positivity, hope, and love. Try it; you might like it. I do about twenty-five minutes of Qigong a day, and Judy and I do another fifteen to twenty minutes of more traditional meditation wrapped in our church-provided prayer shawl.

Well, this gives you some sense of how we are trying to navigate our experiences with Kancer, our wading through conflicting strategies and approaches, and making our decisions.

With appreciation for each of you,
Keith

P.S. For those interested, an anticancer diet includes but is not limited to:

Turmeric

Green Tea (preferably 3 cups a day)

Dark Chocolate (over 70% coca)

Extra Virgin Olive Oil (1st cold press)

Garlic

Only whole grain breads

Only organic, grass-fed meats

Eggs—grass-fed and organic

Fruits

Raspberries, blueberries, stone fruits (e.g. peaches, plums); cherries, avocado

Vegetables (organic)

Asparagus, spinach, yams, broccoli, tomatoes (there is a synergetic anticancer effect when broccoli and tomatoes are eaten together), cabbage (including sauerkraut), Asian mushrooms (such as shitake), cauliflower, beets

4

Framing One's Reality and Plausibility Structures

January 20, 2017

Family, friends,

I am again at the Mayo Clinic, transported here by another che-mo-sabe and receiving a chemo infusion. This treatment is weakened in dosage by 10 percent because my immunity blood count was a bit low—even though my white blood cell count is still strong. In any case, I will have the pack and pump off by midday Sunday, and we will head to Costa Rica that afternoon (Manuel Antonio National Park on the Pacific side for five days).

In two weeks, I will have another CT Scan, and we will see if the tumors have shrunk. I am very convinced that they have. We are doing well. Judy and I are involved in recruiting more than one hundred people from Mayflower Church to attend a meeting/rally with the governor and key legislators to press a justice agenda having to do with immigration policy, mass incarceration, racial equity in education, sustaining the expansion of health care, and other issues. I did a lecture this week on the Theology, Philosophy, and Ethics of Martin Luther King, and I think people enjoyed learning about King as a scholar in the field of philosophy/theology. So we are staying highly engaged and refusing to let cancer determine who we are or what our priorities will be relative to how we spend time and energy.

* * * * * * *

So now is when the nerdy professor begins reflecting on cancer and other matters. I do still receive messages from time to time that my chances of beating this cancer are slim. My parents each survived for a matter of a few months after their cancer diagnoses. How does one sustain hope when messages are contrary to hope and foster cynicism? Today as I receive an infusion to help fight an evil force at the micro level—within my own body—I am well aware that this is inauguration day when a new person takes control of the reigns of the country. I am convinced that this man is not only grossly incompetent; he is evil. He is thoroughly a racist, deeply sexist, Islamophobic, ignorant, narcissistic, vulgar, and hostile to the environment that sustains us. To be honest, I am not at all convinced that democracy can survive this imbecile, and we can only hope that the checks and balances in our system will hold. I am also not at all certain our planet can survive the assault of this man and his cronies: global climate change is real and is at emergency levels. Some people say, "Give him a chance." I have watched this cynical, manipulating, self-serving conman for three decades and have seen him use his wealth and influence to wreak havoc in the lives of many people during those decades. I have also watched him appoint totally incompetent people to many critical positions in the government. Giving him a year to "see what he will do" is about as reasonable as saying, "Keith, let's wait a year before treating this cancer and see what it will do."

So not only is my body under threat; the nation itself is under profound distress. How do we sustain hope in such a time? How do we resist evil—at both the micro and macro levels—when the odds of success seem slim?

This issue of sustaining commitment, hope, and clear vision in the face of countervailing forces is a longtime scholarly interest of mine, and I have found my work in the sociology of religion to be extremely helpful. I have written one piece called "Sustaining Commitment to Teaching in a Cynical World" in which I have applied some of these principles to college teaching: how does one maintain one's spirits and commitment when one gets stabbed in the back by a colleague, an administrator, or even students? That short piece is included at the end of this reflection for those who might be interested. The core issue, however, is sustaining "plausibility structures." Plausibility structures are social and symbolic systems that allow social constructions to seem plausible—even compelling—in spite of contrary evidence (Roberts and Yamane, 2016). People will continue to love, forgive, offer compassion, and stand up for peace, even in the face of overwhelming odds and extraordinary hostility. To do so, however, they need a very strong plausibility structure. *Plausibility structures* are mechanisms that allow one to stay committed to one's better angels and better self, even if it makes one very vulnerable, and even if it defies certain evidence that it is "rational" to do something more self-serving.

All of this has caused me to reflect on what my own plausibility structures are. What sustains my hope and my commitment to resist? What are the social mechanisms that support and sustain my sense of agency?

The *first and most central* component of a plausibility structure is a *community* of people that serve as a reference group. This community is able to affirm and sustain attitudes contrary to the "conventional wisdom." Once a group becomes a powerful reference group, getting together with those people restores one's balance, energizes one for the stressors and "battles" ahead, and re-centers one around the values that one wants to affirm. Our church, my extended family, and an extensive friendship network that has sent notes of encouragement has sustained us in focusing on positive energy and positive imaging. Being surrounded (even if via distance communication) by such people "restoreth my soul." Likewise, being around people in our church and the deeply committed folks at ISAIAH (a consortium of more than one hundred churches working on justice issues in Minnesota) sustains me in resistance to this new president, a manipulator who needs to be *trumped*. So the first and most powerful element of plausibility is a community who holds forth a constructive vision, a hope, and a strategy for moving forward. You have been part of my own plausibility with your support. Plausibility-sustaining communities do not need to be faith communities, but they need to have vision and need to help you be your best self.

Faith communities that have especially strong plausibility structures have not only community but *myths* that sacralize (make sacred) a particular worldview. Myths are stories or narratives that transmit values and perspectives, and they always carry truth. If a myth has no truth to it, it is not a myth; it is merely a fable. Factual accuracy or inaccuracy is not the point of a myth; the truth is in the values and perspectives that they transmit. Narratives of people who have been successful in resistance to cancer (or at the macro level resistance to autocratic leaders) can be deeply sustaining. I have read many such stories and talked to people who have survived cancer (or survived impulsive and erratic autocrats). We need to tell each other success stories that serve as our secular myths to support a worldview for better times. I also find that lot of imaging of a healthy body—and a healthy body politic—serves a kind of mythic role.

Religious groups often reenact myths through *rituals*. Indeed, myths and symbols have a symbiotic relationship with rituals, each contributing to the sacralization of the other. One element of ritual is music, which often makes certain ideas seem so sacred that they are beyond question—they are plausible and compelling. In other instances, music can have a calming effect that allows one to re-center—to remember who one genuinely wants to be. I have found some wonderful harp and/or flute music that complements meditation. Meditating itself is a type of ritual, and I try to spend anywhere from twenty to forty minutes a day in meditation. Some of that is Qigong, which involves hand or body motions that coordinate with certain imagery. Clearly there is a component of ritual in this, and it serves to reinforce a positive social construction of reality for me.

One of the most powerful plausibility structures in faith communities are *symbols*. Edwin Leach once compared a symbol to a computer chip ("Ritualization in Man in Relation to Conceptual and Social Development" in Lessa & Vogt *Reader in Comparative Religion*). Computer chips store a phenomenal amount of information. So do symbols. A cross, for example, has meaning for members of the Christian community because it reminds them of a sacred story, a particular life, a divine event, and the history of a movement. Others

may experience negative memories in relationship to that same symbol, but the symbol delivers much information, and it does so with
powerful emotional content. Whether the symbol is the Star of David,
the eight-spoked wheel, or a national flag, it stores both content and
emotions. I will share one symbol with you that our family is using.
Our niece, Kendra Roberts, makes "wearable art" in New York City
(Kendra Jewelry at http://www.myksj.com/about.php). She has made
for each of the original five K & J Robertses a matching pin or neck-
lace. The one for the men is made from fossilized walrus tusks; the one
for women is similar in appearance but a precious stone. She suggested
that we wear these each day in solidarity—in reminder of the strong
family ties that link us and the incredible family support. It is a very
thoughtful gift, and each of us wears it. I think of my incredible family
support each morning as I put it on.

We have other symbols as well. When I (often with Judy) do a
more traditional Christian—almost Zen—meditation, I or we wrap in
the prayer shawl of our church and are reminded of the support there.
At night, I toss a small blanket from our church in Hanover, Indiana,
over my legs and am reminded of the warmth and support of that community. In each case, the symbol socializes a sense of positive energy
that engulfs me. How can one not be filled with gratitude?

If we hope to resist negative influences that threaten our lives,
and even our social fabric—forces that have great power and seem to
immobilize us—we must cultivate plausibility structures: a supportive
community, myths, rituals, and symbols that cultivate our better angels
and enhance our agency.

Frankly, people will believe all sorts of outrageous things if the
plausibility structures are strong enough—that gods will arrive from
spaceships to save us (Heaven's Gate), that handling poisonous snakes
is part of what is required of Christians and people of faith who handle
them will be protected (snake handling churches of Appalachia), that a
man who died on a cross two thousand years ago is somehow relevant
to us today, or that one should be compassionate and open and vulnerable as a human being or as teachers, even though vulnerable persons
sooner or later are wounded. We all need plausibility structures, or we
become cynical and hardened. We need plausibility structures, or we

lose our sense of agency. That is the "meaning-making" of a sociologist of religion, anyway.

May we all have sustaining plausibility structures that help us to have agency and to resist evil, whether that be at the most micro or the most macro levels of our world. I thank you for ways in which you have been part of my sense of hope and positivity. May we move forward with vigor to a more hopeful, healthy, and compassionate society and world.

Peace and love,
Keith

Sustaining Commitment to Teaching in a Cynical World

Keith A. Roberts
Hanover College

Excellent teaching involves caring, compassion, openness, and accessibility, and it requires significant investment of energy and passion. In short, being a committed and engaged instructor involves an element of vulnerability. When one expends one's energies and tries to be open to others, one is exposed.

The fact is that, sooner or later, virtually every one of us gets wounded. Deans or department chairs may clobber us, colleagues may stab us in the back, students may be apathetic about our beloved discipline and indifferent to our efforts, and other students may trash us in course evaluations. Many students—especially first years—are rational choice theorists who try to get the most reward with the least investment. For us, sociology has meaning—it matters. We seek to construct knowledge in the classroom, and indifference to the process is enervating.

In the face of these situations, it is easy to become cynical—to become negative toward students or to become apathetic toward our institutions. This cynicism, however, stifles excellent teaching. It drains our energies. Continuing to give our best when it is unappreciated seems irrational... even foolish.

Here are two scenarios of this kind of demoralization. In early June, I ran into "Bart"—a really fine colleague who gives his heart, his intellect, and his energies to teaching. I asked him how his summer was going, and he replied, "I am just so glad I do not have to see any students until September. I just read my course evaluations, and the students so completely bludgeoned me that it will take me three months before I can face another class." It turned out that it was actually about a sixth of the class that had said some pretty cruel things, but the negative feedback is often what we take to heart and remember. Bart was so hurt that he needed time to recover before he could teach another class.

A friend of mine from another college had an experience with her administration that took the wind out of her sails. Deb had lined up to be the next faculty member to teach abroad in the college's exchange program. She had planned for months, her husband had arranged to have time off from his work, the family had their passports, and plans for the children to withdraw from the local schools were completed. Deb was really excited, but a few months before they were to leave, the administration notified her that her teaching exchange had been cancelled. She would not be going to Asia. She would have been the first woman to go on this exchange with her family, and it was not clear whether the issue was her gender, or having a family along, or her research agenda. The administration would tell her nothing. She was devastated, demoralized, angry, and enervated by it. She could hardly muster the energy to teach her classes, and she knew she was not at her best in the classroom.

Deb called her close friend and mentor and asked to meet. If anyone could help her recover, it was Janet. They made an appointment, but before they could meet, her key pillar—the person who helped her maintain her spirits when she was down—was killed in an automobile accident. How was she ever going to recover her spirits, regain her commitment to teach in this place she no longer trusted, and give her heart when her efforts were so unsupported and unappreciated?

I have done workshops at professional meetings on combating cynicism, and it has been interesting how nearly every attendee has a story to tell. The specifics vary, but the experience of being demoralized by students, a colleague, or an administrator has been a common one. If cynicism is the first step to burnout and apathy, how do we keep from going there?

In the sociology of religion, scholars have long been interested in how people can continue to believe things that seem improbable and irrational. Why do people continue to affirm that the gods are coming in flying saucers? How is it possible for people to continue to affirm their faith in goodness when they are being abused and tortured by others and their families killed? When a millenarian movement predicts the end of the world, how can people continue to believe the leader after the "expiration date" has already passed? Many do maintain the faith, but only if the "plausibility structures" are strong enough. *Plausibility structures* are social and symbolic systems that allow social constructions to seem plausible—even compelling—in spite of contrary evidence (Roberts and Yamane, 2011; Berger, 1967; Berger and Luchman, 1966). People will continue to love, to forgive, to offer compassion, and to stand up for justice, even in the face of overwhelming odds and extraordinary meanness. To do so, however, they need a very strong plausibility structure.

So maybe what we need in this profession are some plausibility structures that make it seem reasonable to care about our students and our teaching—even if it makes us vulnerable to being hurt again. How can plausibility structures about teaching inoculate us against cynical thinking and negativity?

Plausibility Structures at Work

The first and most central component of a plausibility structure is a *community* of people that become a reference group. This community is able to affirm and sustain attitudes contrary to the "conventional wisdom." Once a group becomes a powerful reference group, getting together with those people restores one's balance, energizes one for the stressors and "battles" ahead, and re-centers one around the values that one wants to affirm. For example, I often create teaching groups of colleagues who care about teaching at my campus. Sometimes we read a book together, or we just talk about teaching issues over a brown bag lunch. The key is to have peers who care about students and have a positive outlook. Being around such people "restoreth my soul."

I also find that I depend on my "fix" of being around teaching-committed people at my regional association meetings and at the ASA Section on Teaching and Learning. Associating with many of the very people who are reading this essay is energizing. I go back in the classroom reaffirming that it makes sense to care and to give my best, even though I may well get clobbered once again. My reference group reminds me that it is "the right thing to do." In short, when my social construction of reality (that teaching really is worth the effort and that it matters) seems in doubt, my teaching friends help that construction to seem plausible and compelling. If you do not have such a community, I recommend that you create one!

Religious communities also have myths that sacralize a worldview. Myths are stories that transmit values and perspectives, and they always carry truth. If a myth has no truth to it, it is not a myth;

it is merely a fable. Factual accuracy or inaccuracy is not the point of a myth; the truth is in the values and perspectives that they transmit. Most of us have stories of transformative learning—either experiences we have had as students or as professional educators. We cherish memories of favorite teachers, and such stories of transformative learning can be inspiring. One can also relive personal moments by maintaining a "feel-good file"—letters and notes sent by students that can be pulled out and reread when needed. Those stories take on a mythical quality by saying, "Yes, the risk-taking does have a benefit; it's worth it."

Religious groups often reenact myths through rituals. Indeed, myths and symbols have a symbiotic relationship with rituals, each contributing to the sacralization of the other. One element of ritual is music, which often makes certain ideas seem so sacred that they are beyond question—they are plausible and compelling. In other instances, music can have a calming effect that allows one to re-center—to remember who one genuinely wants to be. Some faculty find that the last day of a break—before classes start—is a bit of a downer. I have found that I need course preparation rituals the night before the term begins. I focus on the transformative *potential* of the course and listen to music that helps me re-center and become my more humane self. In short, I have rituals that provide an "attitude adjustment." I always seem to enter the class the next day energized, focused, and positive.

One of the most powerful plausibility structures in religious communities are symbols. Edwin

Leach (1972) once compared a symbol to a computer chip. Computer chips store a phenomenal amount of information. So do symbols. A cross, for example, has meaning for members of the Christian community because it reminds them of a sacred story, a particular life, a divine event, and the history of a movement. Others may experience negative memories in relationship to that same symbol, but the symbol delivers much information, and it does so with powerful emotional content. Whether the symbol is the Star of David, the eight-spoked wheel, or a national flag, it stores both content and emotions.

One person I know uses a symbol from the Ecumenical Institute in the 1970s. It is a mathematical symbol, reconstructed here:

This symbol says to this friend: *the past* (on the left) *is not greater than the future* (which he imagines on the right). This reminds him to avoid becoming nostalgic for the "good old days"—when students were supposedly smarter, kinder, more hardworking, and more appreciative. He looks at that symbol before leaving his office to go to class. He refuses to denigrate the current group of students and idealize a former cohort.

Another acquaintance told me that he is intrigued with the sign of the cross. Although the sign is often not made correctly by religious people, it is apparently supposed to involve touching the forehead, the chest, and then both shoulders—the limbs. The idea is that the faith informs how one thinks, how one feels, and how one acts. My acquaintance believes that effective education should engage the mind, the emotions, and ultimately the behavior. Not being especially "religious," he does a truncated version of that sign—touching his forehead, his heart, and one arm before he goes out of his office. It is a reminder that he wants his teaching to be more than short-term memorization. This symbolic act reminds him of his long-standing focus as a teacher.

I mentioned early in this essay that Deb's good friend and mentor was killed in an auto accident right at the time when she especially needed her. It just happened that at precisely that same time, one of her students gave Deb a bracelet. It was one of those WWJD bracelets—which stands for "What would Jesus do?" In the Christian community, it is supposed to remind one to always think of Jesus when making decisions. Deb found that bracelet to be deeply meaningful—though she reconstructed the meaning for the symbol. She would often look at the bracelet in her down moments and think, "What would *Janet* do?" She found it sustaining to remember Janet's deep commitment to students.

I also have a bit of ritual that I use—in connection to a symbol. I have an original linocut by Robert O. Hodgell called *The Professor*. It is a highly satirical image—quite an impersonal and pompous figure pontificating to anyone and to no one. (See photo below.) I stop for five seconds as I go out the door to meet each class, and I remind myself that I do *not* want to look like that—ever! It becomes a negative reminder of what teaching at its worst might look like. It is a bit like touching my head, heart, and limbs as a reminder to be authentic and humane with my students.

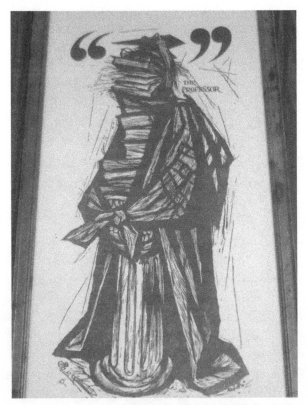

The Professor by Robert O. Hodgell
(www.pchodgell.com/site/)
Used with permission of P. C. Hodgell

If we become cynical, we lose our passion, our commitment, our openness, and our source of energy for teaching each new cohort. Getting stabbed in the back or being kicked in the teeth a few times can quickly foster negativity and cynicism. The antidote is to build some plausibility structures that remind us that students do matter and that we professors are privileged people who get to work with young minds and things of the mind. Reminding myself of this helps me sustain my own commitment to teaching... as I smile through "missing" teeth.

References:

Berger, Peter L. *The Sacred Canopy*. Garden City, N.Y.: Doubleday, 1967.

Berger, Peter L., and Thomas Luckmann. *The Social Construction of Reality*. Garden City, N.Y.: Doubleday, 1966.

Leach, Edmund R. "Ritualization in Man in Relation to Conceptual and Social Development." Pp. 333–37 in *Reader in Comparative Religion*, 3d ed. Edited by William A. Lessa and Evon Z. Vogt. New York: Harper & Row, 1972.

Roberts, Keith A. and David Yamane. *Religion in Sociological Perspective*. 5th edition. Thousand Oaks, CA: SAGE/Pine Forge, 2011.

5

Why Me? Why Us? Micro and Macro Malignancies

February 3, 2017

Family, friends,

It is infusion week again, and this is the time I use to report how I (and we) are doing. Daughter Elise is with me in this private room where I occupy a recliner chair by a sunny window while the staff pumps their poisons into me. Yesterday I also spent the day here at Mayo Clinic, having blood tests, a second CT scan, and a meeting with my oncology team. So there is a bit more to report.

First, the enlarged lymph nodes have shrunk by 50 percent or more. The two largest lung tumors or masses have declined in size by more than 50 percent, and at least one is now "ill-defined." There had been a number of smaller nodules in the lung that have all disappeared. The original malignant mass is in the esophagus, and there is no visible change in the size of that "wall thickening." I was quite surprised by that since I can now swallow foods that I have not previously been able to eat for several months. The doctors said my experience is a better indicator than the imaging, since some of that thickening or mass around the esophagus may well be dead tissue, but they cannot tell that just from the CT scan. The attending oncology nurse practitioner who is part of the team said mine was the most positive report she had given anyone all week.

Two weeks ago, some of my immunity indicators (but not my white blood cell numbers) were low. This time, everything was well within the normal range, and many of the numbers were right in the middle range of normal. The oncology team said my immunity numbers this week were incredibly high. One of the immunity indicators was startlingly strong for someone on chemotherapy.

In short, I am doing well. I have always had energy enough for several people, and I have always felt robust. Well, for about four or five days in the first week after chemo, I must admit I do not feel "robust." My guess is that I feel the way a lot of people feel all the time, but I have never experienced that. I don't feel terrible, but I also do not feel like being the first to volunteer for any and all tasks that come along. It is a lesson in empathy. For those who feel this way—marginal energy a good bit of the time—I wish they could experience what it is like to have really robust health. The second week of my cycle, I feel more like myself and am more inclined to be on the protest lines or testifying at a legislative hearing regarding subtle racism within our social system.

By the way, several people responded to the list of anticancer foods I provided four weeks ago. I should mention that this excellent book, *Anticancer: A New Way of Life* by David Servan-Schreiber, provides lists of anticancer food by specific type of cancer (breast, colon, lung, brain, prostate), and they are somewhat different. So if you are interested in more ideas of foods that are anticancer, do consult that book. It also has a chapter on the cancer-fighting benefits of positive attitudes and of meditation as well as other useful material.

* * * * * * *

Okay, so much for my disease; to me, the more interesting questions are those of meaning-making in a time of personal and social distress. For many people with stage 4 cancer, a common question is "Why me?" As a nation watching someone now in a position of command who has no respect for democracy or for due process, we might also say, "Why us?" Similar to Chronicle 4, I will reflect on both micro (my personal situation) and macro (the nation and global scene). Well, what can I say? I am a sociologist, and we sociologists are always seeing connections between the micro, meso, and macro levels of social life (we call the recognition of the inter linkages the sociological imagination).

So… "Why me?" I guess that sounds a bit like a whiner's question. After all, why not me? Longevity is not "earned," and disease is not a respecter of persons. It happens. It is random. In so far as it is not "just" random, it may be something in my DNA, or something in my environment, or a component of my diet, or a combination of all of these. In any case, the assumption that disease or misfortune should somehow miss me but plague my neighbor is offensive. The underlying assumption that longevity is earned is as offensive as the gospel of prosperity (the theology of our new president). The gospel of prosperity proclaims that the good people will become prosperous and rich, and if one is not prosperous, one is not good. It is a vacuous theology that is as offensive as it is Antichristian (or anti-Jewish and anti-Muslim).

What I am suggesting here is that the very question, "Why me?" that comes so readily to mind is actually a mean-spirited notion that others may deserve this disease, but not me. So I am disinclined to ask that question. I don't deserve to avoid life's troubles any more than the next person. The question is more how we can build a social system that supports any one of us who encounters such "personal troubles"— cancer, or heart trouble, or pervasive hunger, or unemployment, or devastating loss. We are all in this wonderful, rewarding, difficult, painful, exhilarating experience of life together and need to pay attention to the *common* good—a resource *to* which we all should contribute and *from* which we can draw as needed. I have cancer—stage 4 cancer to be more specific—but I have phenomenal support, incredible medical care at Mayo and via alternative treatments, and the resources (including health insurance) that many people do not have. It may seem odd to say, "I have cancer," *and* "I am blessed," all in the same breath, but it is true. Send your helpful, positive energies and images my way, for they are healing, but direct no pity my way, for it would be misdirected.

So, why us? Well, why not? In many ways, we face a truly serious threat to democracy, and that threat is directly related to the threat many of us may well be facing at the micro level with "personal troubles." While we were in Costa Rica last week, I read Henry Giroux's *America at War With Itself*, a truly remarkable little book. Giroux holds the professorship for scholarship in the Public Interest and the Paulo Freire Distinguished Scholar Chair in Critical Pedagogy at McMaster University, and he has the most focused and insightful analysis of why we now have Trump as president of anything I have seen. The book was published last spring when the Republican primaries were not entirely decided, but his discussion of Trump is prescient. The words *Trump*, *totalitarian*, and *tyranny* are far more than alliterative—they absolutely belong together; but the move toward authoritarian or totalitarian rule is more than a one-person phenomenon. It has been building for at least a couple of decades in the United States, and while many of us have been alarmed by specific issues or developments, I, for one, had failed to see the overriding pattern that he describes. That pattern is well documented by renowned political scientists, historians, rhetoricians, and economists who have studied the rise of dictatorships and totalitarianism across time and in many parts of the world.

These features identified by Giroux—the forerunners of tyranny—include (but are not limited to):

a) extreme expressions and celebrations of patriotism at otherwise neutral events like professional and college sports;

b) lionization of soldiers, including constant reference to soldiers as our heroes on nightly news, and nearly obligatory expressions of thanks for their service on airplanes and in stores;

c) celebration of military action or other uses of force as the solution for nearly every problem with the implicit understanding that war is a good rather than always an evil (perhaps sometimes a necessary evil but still an evil);

d) embracing of torture, the most heinous of human rights abuses and one of the least effective methods of interrogation;

e) demonization, objectification, and pathologizing of persons with disabilities;

f) demonization of immigrants and fear-mongering relative to all people of color ("otherizing" them);

g) challenging women's rights, their value to society affirmed pretty exclusively as sex objects and procreators;

h)   undermining of public education through standardized testing that focuses on rote memorization and uniform methodologies rather than students learning to interpret, analyze, synthesize, and even generate meanings as critical thinkers and deep learners;

i)   generating great fear about people's safety—the "real" people that is, those who are white and privileged;

j)   creating "alternative facts" (fictions) to support a particular agenda and narrative regarding who we are and where we are headed;

k)   abdicating by media of its essential role of holding public officials and office seekers accountable and simultaneously confusing "fair and balanced" coverage as including all points of view as valid, even if some arguments are clearly specious and contrary to empirical evidence (facts);

l)   normalizing self-interest as the best and perhaps only motive for any behavior [and of course, *all* right wing policy is premised on the core principle that everyone must pursue his or her self-interests, and we must make people feel pain (more cost than benefit) if they behave in ways that are contrary to the best interests of the larger society (as determined by the financial elite)]; and

m)   fostering close adherence to neoliberalism in framing all social policies. Neoliberalism stresses the privatization of many government functions, lauding individualism above the common good, and reduction of the public square (where ideas can be debated by the people) in favor of think tanks like ALEC (the American Legislative Exchange Council) that create and spread policies that benefit the already wealthy and privileged.

Although many of Trump's assertions and policies are, as both republican Ohio governor John Kasich and democratic Maryland governor Martin O'Malley said, deeply connected to Nazi rhetoric, Trump totalitarianism will have its own flavor and unique dimensions quite different from the Nazi programs of Germany. Still, we must recognize both Trump's focus and the overall trend of the country as toward a more autocratic, authoritarian, and antidemocratic milieu. Note for example that some presidents (of both parties, including Obama) have turned to executive orders in frustration when Congress seemed immobilized by gridlock. No president of this country, however, has ever *begun* his presidency with "governance by executive order." If you did not see it, the editorial "The Republican Fausts" by conservative *New York Times* columnist David Brooks on January 31, 2017 was excellent and worth reading (https://www.nytimes.com/2017/01/31/opinion/the-republican-fausts.html?_r=0).

All of this is not to say that Trump will not have some positive impacts and successes. As a sociologist who has taught courses focusing on policy analysis, I well know that all policies have unexpected consequences. Policies that sound great often have some unfortunate side effects, and policies that appear to be disasters in the making sometimes have some pluses we had not anticipated. I am well aware that many First Nations peoples—especially those in the Southwest—celebrate Richard Nixon's birthday every year and consider him to be by far the best president this country has ever had. This adulation is for a man who tried to sabotage the constitution and was clearly a crook, but he is the only president to return sacred land (Blue Lake in New Mexico) to indigenous peoples (the Taos). Likewise, one of the world's most brutal and corrupt dictators the world has ever known—Rafael Trujillo of the Dominican Republic—was the most progressive environmentalist the world has ever known as a head of state. My assumption is that even totalitarian Trump will do some things that have positive outcomes (even if those outcomes are unintended). We need to watch for and celebrate those moments when light does break through, and the moral arc of the universe takes a bend toward justice (as MLK would say).

In the meantime, our private troubles are likely to be ignored and unsupported at the macro levels in a climate that celebrates the privatization of everything public; the demeaning of a sense of the common good in favor of radical individualism; issuing of executive orders that further privileges of whites, males, Euro-Americans; and legislative initiatives that foster a "survival of the fittest" ethos and favor the rich. We must be committed and push beyond private troubles to public concerns, which affect us all. I plan to fight like hell for my health against this malignancy that has invaded my body, but I also pledge to resist the malignancy that has overtaken our country. I do not just mean the idiocy of this forty-fifth president but also the larger cultural patterns that have delivered us to his doorstep. I am comforted to know that so many of you are also stepping beyond personal troubles to work for a more humane, caring, compassionate, and just social system that can nourish us all. Yet—Geez—it is such a big task.

My mother was a popular inspirational public speaker, especially with church and civic groups. She had one metaphor she used on many occasions that I think fits our situation. It seems that in the 1950s, General Electric was trying to stress the power of individuals who had resilience and abiding determination. In their headquarters, GE hung a one-ton steel ball by a very long chain from a ceiling a couple of stories up. Then they had a one- or two-ounce cork—like we used to use as bobbers when fishing as kids—and had it coordinated to swing with a rhythm into the side of that steel ball. The timing of the cork had to be done strategically, but within two weeks, that one-ton ball began to move—just barely. The cork had to be adjusted so its "hammering" timed with the movement of the ball, but within a month or six weeks, that ball was moving six inches to a foot. Eventually, the ball was swinging more than that in a regular rhythm, rather like a pendulum on a clock. Sometimes when we are trying to bring change to macro systems (even when we are trying to change something in our private lives), it feels like we are beating our heads against a one-ton steel ball. But I believe that is what we are called to do. We are to be the corks, getting that immoveable "heavy" mass to swing toward something better, something constructive, something ultimately healthy and redeeming. It is hard work and sometimes demoralizing, but it is not just one cork at work; it is thousands of us working in concert. There is hope if we do not give up hope. There can be movement toward the good if we—collectively—insist on it. First, we must not dwell on, "Why me?" regarding our private troubles and instead look for that steel ball and strategize with others about how to get it moving! Micro healing and macro healing are linked, and I (we) must keep that fact in focus. We must never focus on only one level.

Peace and love,
Keith

6

Faith, Values, and Healing

February 17, 2017

Family, friends,

I am again at the Mayo Clinic attached to intravenous tubes for infusion. Not much new to report medically this week since I did not see a doctor. Folks whom I encounter at church and other contexts keep telling me that I look terrific, though the guy I see in the mirror looks pretty much like a flesh-covered skeleton to me. Lots of folks in my age cohort keep saying that "they just don't make things like they used to." Perhaps that especially applies to mirrors—the ones they make nowadays just don't give a good reflection. There is some old geezer in my mirror, not me! In any case, the scales are also telling me I weigh about what I did when I was a sophomore in high school—though I don't feel quite ready to try high jumping, running high hurdles, or relishing the challenge of guarding a center four inches taller than myself on the basketball court. Actually, in the past five days, I have gained about six pounds back, so I am finally moving in the right direction.

On the other hand, I am feeling good most of the time. Judy and I are attending justice rallies and community-organizing events, so we are active and involved. I do occasionally have something catch in my esophagus—behind the sternum. I am now eating things I have not tried to eat for three or four months, but the "thickening of the walls" of the esophagus has not diminished. Although this thickening may be largely dead tissue now, it is problematic at times, so that is a focus of my own prayer/meditation time.

I have said that we are approaching this health crisis with multi-faceted strategies, but I have had some queries that I be more specific. I am doing all of the following, and my assumption is that these are complementary and synergetic. So we utilize:

- Chemotherapy (every other week; part of this is a drug targeted specifically at my HER2 marker);
- Diet adjustments (for example, every effort to avoid processed cane or beet sugar and trying to eat more anticancer foods) combined with supplements that naturopathy specialists recommend for anticancer health;
- Qigong and Qi-ssage (the latter involves full body massages focused on acupressure points; alternate weeks)
- Healing touch energy treatments (opposite weeks of the Qi-ssage);
- Personal daily meditation (20–40 minutes per day);
- Various faith-community prayer groups from around the country that direct healing my direction;
- Aroma therapy (our daughter has given us an aroma therapy steamer and frankincense—which seems to me to be premature embalming, but what do I know?);
- Shamanistic healing exercises/rituals performed by cousins trained by an indigenous healer in Peru;
- Exercise (daily stationary bike workouts, along with some other activities);
- Social activism (more on why this is a healing strategy below).

I do have one health issue I will need to address in coming weeks. My Mayo medical team said two weeks ago that *after* this round of four treatments (my eighth infusion), we will do another CT scan and hopefully see still further reduction of the tumors. At that point, they may decide to keep up the medication targeting the HER2, but I would take a break from the other chemo. One reason for the break would be that I have developed a hernia, and I must be off of chemo for one month before I can undergo hernia repair, and a second month after the surgery before chemo can be resumed. Here is the dilemma: the doctor said we may cut the chemo and go to a "maintenance regimen." Although I have known all along that with stage 4 cancer there is only a 1-percent chance of cure, I still have hope of such an outcome. I think the doctors see cure so very rarely that they do not really have cure on their radar. This is palliative treatment. I did not like the sound of "maintenance regimen." At what point is it wise to insist on pushing the envelope for cure, and at what point is this insistence just living in denial? That is a question for which an answer seems illusive. I keep thinking of Reinhold Niebuhr's now famous prayer (often misattributed to "anonymous"): "God, grant me the serenity to live with those things that cannot be changed, the courage to change those things that can be changed, and the wisdom to distinguish the one from the other." (This is the actual wording of the original prayer). That is what I lack right now: wisdom relative to this diagnosis. Please understand that for me, finding that this cancer cannot be cured (if that should be the case) does not mean acquiescence. I think there is still a fight for longevity and for quality of life that can both be won, even if cancer is not eradicated from my body. Yet the ideal scenario is for it to be vanquished entirely, and as of right now, that is still the goal.

* * * * * * *

Well, I have already begun the discussion of making meaning of the situation we face. Much of my writing for the last two sessions have focused on dual resistance: micro against cancer and macro against a truly sinister and buffoonish clown who has seized power in this country and is a real threat to democracy. I have one or two people who thought my comments are "political," but I do not regard them as "political" at all. I regard my remarks as commentaries on *social ethics*, which was a major focus of much of my graduate work. Moreover, after forty years of teaching critical, analytical thinking, I am convinced that this president is not even sophomoric in his demeanor and presentation of self. His analytical skills are so truncated and underdeveloped that I have *rarely* had a college first-year student so lacking in basic thinking skills. We have elected a mental—and moral—minnow. However, I do not wish to focus further on this saboteur of democracy. Rather, I would reflect on why the condition of the country might matter to someone facing a life-threatening disease.

When I was in college, I had the privilege to hear Viktor Frankl speak, and he—a survivor of Holocaust death camps—said pointedly to us, "Never seek happiness in life, or you will miss the mark. Happiness is not a goal to be pursued but a side product of something else. If you seek to engage in meaningful activity and lead a meaningful life, something far deeper than happiness will be with you—even if you are in the most hopeless of situations. Seek meaning, and happiness and hope and contentment arrive as byproducts." I have found his advice to be sage wisdom, indeed. Interestingly, when Judy and I were married, my brother, Bruce, performed the ceremony and delivered the homily; his message was that having a common goal—a meaningful shared focus—is a stronger glue to a marriage than just pouring attention on each other. So it is that focusing on a common goal—a just, compassionate, and sustainable social order—that is part of my (and our) mission in life, part of my therapy, part of my being. So I hope that my sharing of this worldview is not just self-indulgent on my part but provides a larger vision of what it means to be fully human. In addition, meaningful work to create a more just world is deeply healing. Having a purpose is invigorating and restorative to both body and soul (Dali Lama and Desmond Tutu, *The Book of Joy*).

Most of you know that I consider myself a person of faith, but I have never really understood *faith* as having much of anything to do with *beliefs*. That, to me, is a trivialization of faith. Faith is absolutely *not* about ideas one holds in one's head or about creeds or dogma. John Wesley liked to say that faith is not about creeds but about deep relationships—both vertical and horizontal. Martin Luther King, Jr. liked to quote his Boston University mentors in saying that "the moral arc of the universe is long, but it bends toward justice." That is not so much a "belief" as a deeply held orientation to life and to the larger world in which we live; it is a framing about how one perceives the world. My faith calls me to be a participant in that bending, to help create a world of compassion, humaneness, justice, and love. Faith is expressed less by ideas in one's head than by actions one takes and the way one lives out a life. So the core to "faith" for me is that it is the organizing principle of how one actually lives. Its manifestation is a life of integrity. The question for someone like me at this stage in life is how does one live a consistent life focused on the good when a major *distraction* (cancer) enters the scene?

So my healing focus at the micro level is that I refuse to be defined by "cancer"—to let that somehow take priority in how I live and how I relate to the world around me. I refuse to give it that much power over my life. So Judy and I move forward, slowed and sometimes detoured by this ailment but seeking meaningful engagements. Next week, we gather with dear, dear friends—a group of twelve of us who were part of a small group in a Newton, Massachusetts, church in the early '70s. We meet for three days every other year, and so we continue to deepen this supportive set of relationships. This time, we meet in Los Cruces, New Mexico. After that, Judy and I fly to Alaska to see granddaughter Adina (and we might even say hi to our son and daughter-in-love). Meanwhile, I am planning to teach an OLLI (Osher Lifelong Learning Institute) course on religion and social inequality (the links connecting religion to racism, sexism, classism, and heterosexism) in the spring. In addition, I am organizing a tour of sacred Dakota grounds in the Twin Cities in the summer. We are also deeply engaged in work in the Twin Cities relative to racial inequities in schools, mass incarceration of people of color in this state, the sanctuary movement and other actions on behalf of immigrants, and efforts to stop predatory profiteering (such as the payday lending scams that are underwritten by U.S. Bank and other lending institutions).

Am I just in denial about my own actual health crisis? I prefer to think I am just living life meaningfully and to its fullest. Life is good! That can also be true of life in the shadow of cancer! Indeed, life is good. This is expressed so eloquently in a Kaddish read at the funeral of a Mayflower Church friend—Larry Turner. May we each leave a legacy like this when we finally depart.

Mourner's Kaddish
by Merrit Malloy

When I die give what's left of me away
to children and old men that wait to die.
And if you need to cry,
cry for your brother walking the street beside you.
And when you need me, put your arms around anyone
and give them what you need to give me.

I want to leave you something,
something better than words or sounds.
Look for me in the people I've known or loved,
and if you cannot give me away
at least let me live in your eyes and not in your mind.

You can love me best by letting hands touch hands,
and by letting go of children that need to be free.
Love doesn't die, people do.
So, when all that's left of me is love,
give me away.

Peace and love,
Keith

7

Paradigms and Constructions of Reality

March 6, 2017

Family, friends,

Infusion day means Kancer Chronicle writing, and this is that day. I have felt great over the past two weeks with no nausea and energy levels high. I was, therefore, surprised when the doctor told me my immunity indicators, especially my neutrophil (white blood cell) count was down. We still did an infusion but with another reduction in strength of treatment (down 25 percent from the original dose), so I do have to get those immunity system numbers back up. If they drop any further, they will cancel my next infusion. The other less positive development is that I am again having food "catch" behind the sternum, which is quite painful. I also have to have another echocardiogram to monitor my heart. In another month, we will have a CT scan to see how I am doing with shrinking those tumors any further. It is common for people on the chemo regimen I am on to experience some neuropathy, but I have had very little of that.

Our son, Kent, is now settled in his own apartment about five blocks from us, and we will see Justin and his family in Alaska this Saturday, so we are surrounded by family in addition to incredible support from others around us and around the country.

* * * * * * *

In my last Chronicle, I said that I am a person of faith but that I do not think that faith is about "beliefs"; faith is much deeper than beliefs. I received some reactions to that and queries asking for more explanation. This all has to do with finding or creating meaning, so it seems relevant to what I am doing in these Kancer chronicles.

Beliefs are ideas that we hold in our heads. However, many, perhaps most, beliefs have little impact on our actual behavior or our lived values. One interesting example is the survey (some years ago now) showing that among people who "believe very strongly" in the Ten Commandments, only 40 percent could name more than two of them, and only about 10 percent could list more than eight. This was among people who were "strong believers" in those principles. What does it mean to believe in something one cannot even identify by name? Likewise, a very substantial percentage of North Americans who agree that all humans are children of God also indicate high levels of prejudicial altitudes toward blacks and various ethnic minorities.

I would suggest that the relationship between faith and belief is much like the relationship between a value and a velleity. Suppose that we ask a man if he values reading. He may respond that reading is very worthwhile and is important to him. In a forced-choice questionnaire, he may rate reading more highly than television, and he may agree with the statement, "Daily reading should be a part of every adult's life." He can wax eloquently on reading and really does hold this conviction with some intensity. Yet we may find that this same fellow spends two or three hours per evening watching television and that he has not read a book for several years, *rarely* reads substantive journals or magazines, and looks only at headlines in his daily newspaper. We might conclude, contrary to his verbal insistence, that he really values reading very little. His behavior suggests that television has priority on his time. Reading is not so much a *value* as a *velle*ity. This fellow would like reading to be a value, but in the actual scheme of things, he does not act on his feeling of ought. Stevens concludes, "A velleity is something I would like, but I'm not prepared to act on it. A value is something I consistently act upon. Action is the acid test of value" (*The Morals Game*. New York: Paulist Press. 1974: 13–14). So when we are talking about a value, it involves walking the talk.

Likewise, I would argue that faith is what is one's actual "center of value" (worth-ship) and the core organizing principle(s) of one's life—even if those are not totally conscious to the person. The acid test of faith is action. It is actually lived and manifested in all substantive decisions one makes. If a notion about life is not enacted in everyday life, it is not "faith." The phrase from Martin Luther King that "the moral arc of the universe is long, but it bends toward justice" was not just words or ideas in his head; it was something that he knew deep in his bones to be true, and it animated his struggle for "the beloved community." Faith is sometimes only semiconscious. That is why when I was in seminary, Hebrew Bible scholar Harrell Beck often suggested that if we want to have clarity about our faith rather than scrutinize the ideas in our heads, we would do better to do a content analysis of our checkbooks, for the expenditures of our bank account may well be a stronger indicator of what has priority in our lives than our "beliefs." Sometimes we may be surprised at what has actually been at the core of our decision-making and has been our priority.

So are beliefs always ephemeral, shallow, and insignificant? Not at all. In essay #4, I talked about how very important plausibility structures are: a community that reaffirms a worldview and set of values plus symbols, myths (beliefs), and rituals that help to sacralize our worldview. We must have plausibility structures to keep us focused on those values and principles that in our deepest moments of reflection we know to be true (even if we waver in the stresses of everyday life). Some beliefs really are superficial and are more words than real convictions, but other beliefs are deeply held and are part of our plausibility structures—the myths, symbols, and rituals that sustain our faith in the face of deep challenges. So beliefs can be terribly important, and they can sometimes cause us to realign or rethink our faith, but they are not the same thing as "faith."

In one sense, faith is the lens through which one sees and makes sense of the world. My "lens" has been informed by my experiences in the church and family regarding the meaning of life, but it has also been shaped by my deep commitment to empiricism as a scientist—a sociologist. For the most part, those lenses have been highly congruent. In sociology, two of the important paradigms or overarching theoretical paradigms are rational choice perspective and social constructionism. These Kancer chronicles are deeply informed and shaped by the social construction paradigm.

Rational choice theory, which is at the core of most economic theory, views humans as always pursuing their self-interests. Humans are basically incapable of genuine altruism, for every action is assessed in terms of costs and benefits to the individual. Moreover, while humans are rational in calculating costs and benefits, they are not seen as particularly self-reflective or active as meaning makers. Indeed, individuals are reactive to these choices rather than proactive in defining reality and, therefore, have limited agency. Virtually all conservative social policy is based on a rational choice view of human behavior. Conservatives are often characterized as "mean-spirited," for conservative social policies try to control unwanted behavior by increasing the cost and, thereby, deterring that behavior by changing the pleasure/pain ratio. Whether the policy is designed to deter out-of-wedlock pregnancies, immigration, homicide, theft, burglary, or white-collar crime, the solution is always the same—*increase the pain* for the unwanted behavior and enhance the rewards for the desired behavior. Conservatives dismiss liberals as bleeding hearts, for liberals think with their hearts rather than their heads: they lessen the pain by providing supports for single-parent parents, immigrants, or even law breakers. This, they say, will just result in more of the unwanted behavior. (*In some cases*, conservatives are correct about that.) Even the God of those holding to this rational choice paradigm is one who punishes people (either here and now or in the afterlife) if they do not obey God's commandments. Imposition of pain is the core mechanism for conservative social policy and other behavioral controls.

By contrast, social constructionism suggests that humans are meaning-constructing animals. We humans constantly try to figure out what things mean, we use symbols to help us understand the reality around us, and we are active agents in creating meaning when meaning is ambiguous. We are self-reflecting beings that often seek to be guided by values and ideals, and we may well act contrary to our narrow individual self-interests if we believe it is the right thing to do in creating a beloved and just community. (Martin Luther King, Jr., who had a sociology major in college, was a social constructionist, and his systematic theology departed from much Christian "orthodoxy" as he tried to formulate a theology that made sense of the black experience.)

Persons often seek integrity as a self-seeking consistency between our worldview and our actions. We may well choose to define reality in line with only personal pleasure/pain ratio, but that is a variable—a choice—rather than an unbending rule or drive of all human behavior. Social polices based on this social constructionism paradigm see persons as actively creating meaning and actively defining reality. In terms of social policy, it often tries to help "deviants" to redefine their own role in the social system. Emphasis on *rehabilitation* rather than more draconian, *painful penalties* is one manifestation of this difference.

According to the construction model, we humans are proactive in designing our lives, our social arrangements, and our values for making decisions. In light of this, many persons of faith stress an *alternative reality* to the punitive one so common in the larger culture, emphasizing instead ideas like grace, compassion, distributive justice, and taking the perspective of the "other."

As a person immersed in both a theologically progressive Christian community and the empiricism of the social sciences, social constructionism resonates deeply and shapes the way I define reality. I struggle to make sense of my cancer in ways that affirm my own agency, emphasize reason and logic in forming a coherent view of life, validate the role of the heart, and open me always to new insights and to the experience of others. This, to me, is part of being a person of faith. When I write that I reject the notion that "stage 4 cancer" is a synonym for "terminal cancer" (they need not be the same thing!) or that Judy and I *refuse to be defined by cancer* and give it power in our lives, I am using a constructionist paradigm to define our reality. This is challenging since a "stage 4 cancer diagnosis" has a way of never being far from one's consciousness, and I need plausibility structures to keep my alternative definition of reality strong and central. These chronicles are an effort to create meaning in an ambiguous and perhaps threatening situation. I write with hope that they provide a window on meaning for others, and I write with a deep appreciation for the way in which many of you have helped shape my own social constructions of "reality." You continue to be part of my alterative plausibility structure. Whether I ultimately prevail over this cancer or not, I live in the meantime with hope and positive energy—directed toward creating a beloved community.

Peace and love,
Keith

8

Living with Ambiguity

March 20, 2017

Family, friends,

Infusion day again. With a trip to Alaska in the midst of this two-week period, it feels from here like this has been a short time between chronicles. I have been feeling good and have good energy. Son Justin felt I had much more energy—for things like participating in a Lubavitcher (Hasidic Jewish) Purim event in Anchorage—than I had in December. I just got a report that my immunity indicators are back up in the normal range, and an echocardiogram early this morning indicates my heart is strong and not affected by the chemo. I am doing better with food passing through the esophagus but still have an occasional glitch. Even the "glitches" are less painful than they have been in the past. I do know that my overall strength is down, and I am often aware of "pressure" in the middle of my chest (pain would be too strong of a word, but discomfort is experienced). Still, given the stunning surprise diagnosis of less than four months ago, I am active and involved. We attended the dedication of infant Quinn Gilbert Conkle yesterday, followed in the evening by a concert by the Earth Justice composer, Jim Scott. Tomorrow I will be at the state capital for a rally and hearing objecting to the opening of a privatized prison in this state, and next week, I begin a class I am teaching on religion and social inequality. So all things considered, I have no major complaints.

* * * * * *

So what are the issues of meaning-making that I have been reflecting on most recently? I do think one of the challenges for people with a chronic, life-threatening disease is *ambiguity*. I am struck with how much of our living is now constrained by, shaped by, and/or responsive to ambiguity. We hope that healing is occurring, but it is unseen. We hope the healing is so complete that it is actually a *cure*, but we know the odds are slim on that count. Healing can occur in ways that fall short of cure, so being in remission for some years is healing but without full "cure." This sort of healing is wonderful in itself, but of course, one then lives knowing the cancer still is dormant in one's body and can reassert itself at any point, blindsiding one at a later date. Yes, ambiguity becomes a constant companion when one has an ailment like cancer. It is never very far from consciousness and certainly has a "hand" on one side of the scales whenever one contemplates decisions about the future or tries to make plans.

In *Letters from the Land of Cancer*, Walter Wangerin writes, "A serious disease invades more than the body's physical symptoms." Indeed, it is true. He continues, "It invades by creating an entire meteorology of disturbances... What it disturbs and tests is... the rest of me: my character, personality, faith, morality, virtue, the spirit's gifts as well as the spirit's vacuities" (p. 113). The destructive meteorological vortex within has the potential to hurt those around me if my moods swing, I am unappreciative, or I allow the negativity within to leak out and infect others. Judy tells me that since my diagnosis, I smile much less than I used to, that in my relaxed state around the house my mouth tends to fall at the edges rather than rise. Much of the spinning storm within me is related to ambiguity (though I must say that with the sinister buffoon running the administrative branch of the national government, there are plenty of other things contributing to a permanent frown). Disease invades the body (or grows through abnormal mutations from within); this brings ambiguity in many areas of life decisions, resulting in a churning, or even an inner hurricane.

Wangerin comments that "when we are young, we strive forward, peering toward and planning for better things to come. But we based the forward presumptions of our forward-peering-planning on the experiences of our past, such as getting sick and getting better every time" (p. 115). However, with stage 4 cancer or other major chronic

60

disease, the calculus—the process—of thinking about the future and planning one's life suddenly changes. "One gets sick and then does not get better again. A fellow finds himself boxed in: fewer future years, fewer promises to be drawn from all those many former years" (p. 138). In terms of planning even for near future like the fall, do we schedule that trip to Greece we always wanted to take—perhaps with Road Scholar doing the organizational work for us? What will my treatment regime be by then, and how will my energy levels hold up? Will my esophagus handle the foods that are provided by the planners? (I cannot eat any meats, but soft ones—fish and very tender or ground meats—and spicy dishes drive my esophagus crazy.) For the fall, should I offer an eight-week Osher Lifelong Learning course, which I so thoroughly enjoy doing? What do we not yet know about this cancer journey and where it will take us in six months?

Wangerin suggests that the solution to the forward-peering-planning conundrum is twofold: continue to plan for those things that really are meaning-filled—things that really matter—and "spiritually to approach [one's] losses with the same craft and talent and devotion to which one has [approached one's vocation or other beloved tasks]" (p. 139). Can this old dog learn to approach losses of activities and possible longevity and acceptance of ambiguity with that kind of focused commitment? It is a formidable challenge. Not doing things because of the cancer is to give it too much power in my life, but realistically I do know that the cancer delimits some of my options.

How does one do this? How does one keep the inner storm and ambiguity from disturbing those closest whom one loves? First is to acknowledge that they probably also have a kindred storm within. I am not at all sure I am helping either Judy or my three kids with their inner storms. What could I be doing better? I am hoping that others in our supportive community are helping them, and I do believe that they are. Judy, for example, now has a "befriender" from the church who is a supportive, listening ear. Judy has to face every bit as much ambiguity as I, and plans for her and our futures are impacted as the forward-peering-planning calculus is suddenly different for her.

Few people like ambiguity, and some people go to extremes to avoid it—accepting rigid and narrow literalistic religious interpretations of Scripture and of dogma, for example. One will even give up his or her God-given freedom of thought to escape ambiguity. Yet ambiguity is not escapable. One must find ways of accepting and living with it. Indeed, there are few greater dangers to civilization than those ideologues who are unable to cope with ambiguity—especially if the ambiguity-avoidant ideologues have power.

I do think that I see three major realms of ambiguity in my own life that may be models of living constructively with ambiguity, though these have been less intimate than this malignant invasion of my body. One model comes from my role as a (social) scientist. Many nonscientists think that science offers truth with a capital T and seeks certainty. Nothing could be further from reality. Any good scientist knows that she or he accepts any theory tentatively. Future research may well undermine a current theory and cause a new paradigm to emerge that better explains the data. Moreover, scientific research is typically set up in a way that can *disprove* what one believes to be true—one's hypothesis. If the research cannot disprove the hypothesis or theory, then that becomes more data in support of the explanation. However, no good scientist ever says he or she has "proved" something. That is too strong of causal language for a dynamic enterprise like science. There are always new variables to be tested and new ways to frame the problem. So ongoing ambiguity is a constructive reality in science, including the social sciences.

One must move forward with the best knowledge that we have at the time, and one must trust the empirically validated facts as the strongest basis for deliberations about policy or future decisions. However, there is always an awareness that what we know is incomplete and subject to future discoveries. Truth is not buried in the *past*—ensconced in sacred scriptures (even though those scriptures may offer valuable wisdom). Further, truth is not something revealed in full by a charismatic leader in the *past*. Truth is a result of triangulation of new findings and insights of empirical sciences that is informed by reason (logic), experience, and wisdom. So truth will be greater in the *future* than in the past. One moves forward with the best evidence and conclusions we have to date—the *preponderance of the evidence*. In the case of the overwhelming evidence for climate change, the lives of our grandchildren may depend on *immediate intervening action*, so lack of absolute proof cannot be grounds for inaction. Thus, as a scientist, I have learned to embrace ambiguity as a positive reality as part of the challenge of seeking truth and good social policy. Indeed, social policy itself always has unexpected, unanticipated consequences (both constructive and destructive), so it always has some ambiguity.

A second source of ambiguity, interestingly, is faith itself. To cite one of many excellent treatments of faith, Paul Tillich stresses in *Dynamics of Faith* that faith and doubt are not opposites at all, that they are closely linked partners in the lifelong search for meaning and purpose. In a church Judy and I attended, I once heard an associate pastor comment in a sermon about a faith practice, concluding, "I guarantee that if you [do this], your life will be richer." I wondered first at what the guarantee was—that my contribution to the offering plates would be refunded? I also was appalled that any theologically trained person could speak with such absolutes and such certainty. Faith involves wisdom in shaping one's life around core organizing principles or values, but those are convictions. One is willing to stake one's life on those values rather than another set of values. It is a bet-my-life-on-it framing of what gives existence on this planet meaning and purpose. There are no absolute certainties; there is commitment to a greater vision in the midst of ambiguity, and even doubt. This is at the core of what faith means. So as a person of faith, I have tried to always see the positive sides of ambiguity. (It can be a challenge, but it is important.)

Third, as an activist and sociologist committed to a just and compassionate society, I find myself faced with a demagogue—a mean-spirited maniac—shaping the policies of the nation in which I live and of which I am a citizen. I worked hard, and we contributed thousands of dollars to political campaigns this past year, but we ended up with an ignorant sinister boor as president and both chambers of congress controlled by a party complicit in his rise and his hold on power. Franky, I think it is an open question whether democracy can survive; he has systematically initiated all of the major steps that tyrannical dictators around the world have used—including undermining the courts and the press that should *serve* as checks and balances on any authoritarian leader. (An excellent analysis of this is an interview of Erica Chenoweth, a leading scholar on authoritarian regimes and how to resist them in *The Nation* at https://www.thenation.com/article/how-to-topple-a-dictator/.) Hopefully, the checks and balances built into our system are strong enough to resist this would-be autocrat, and it may well be (says political scientist Jake Smith) that one of our best hopes is the often vilified bureaucracy in our government, for public employees in the U.S. government can be masters of slow-things-down-so-nothing-gets-done resistance. It may well be the much-maligned federal bureaucratic structure that saves us. How is that for irony? However, we cannot depend on that. We *must* resist both the mean-spirited policies and the sinister attempts to undermine the structures that ensure democracy. His current 37 percent approval rating is extraordinarily low this early in a presidency, and that is encouraging, as it will lessen support for him among politicians within his own party. In any case, we live in highly dangerous and very ambiguous times politically. The ambiguity in this case is whether or not we can stop Herr Trump. It is also true that it is very likely that Trump will do some things—even if unintentionally—that are positive for the country, and it is important to recognize this. No president in history has been without both horrible mistakes and constructive contributions, so our ambiguity also calls for some humility at times. Any good activist must recognize and live constructively with ambiguity. Ambiguity is often the catalyst for deeper commitment.

Learning in my lifetime to embrace ambiguity may prove to be a huge asset. So the question is, can I transfer this knowledge so that ambiguity can be constructive to the more intimate matter of ambiguity about my health, and even my life? I have certainly not mastered that yet. I *am* convinced that having strong plausibility structures (discussed in essay #4) is one key to a positive attitude and constructive coping. I am trying to deal with ambiguity—which is likely to be a presence, a given for the rest of my life. I am trying to make it a friendly adversary and perhaps a source of personal growth. This involves a social construction of reality and seizing agency in creating meaning. If I can change my attitude toward the many ambiguities I face—healing versus living in a sick role, longevity versus rather early demise, forward-looking living versus the prospect of diminished future, unknowns about health and energy levels at every turn—perhaps what I experience will be a less violent vortex and instead be an earth and air cleansing thundershower.

Am I a naive fool? Perhaps, but it seems to be a path that has integrity and potential for positive relationships and positive energy in facing this health challenge. It may be the best strategy to make sure the disease of my body does not seep into a disease of my spirit, a healthy spirit being essential to a healing body.

In two weeks, I have another CT scan, and some ambiguity about my physical condition/progress may be temporarily relieved.

So much for my meaning-making in these past two weeks. I hope your own lives are filled with meaning and meaning-making.

Peace and love,
Keith

9

How Do I Name This Experience? Warlike and Non-warlike Metaphors

April 3, 2017

Family, friends,

Greeting from Infusion Land, Mayo Clinic, MN. I will have four hours connected to IVs, so it is a good time to write. Three days ago (Friday), I spent the day here at Mayo with various tests, including a third CT scan. My blood tests indicate healthy immunity systems. In late January (eight weeks ago), the CT scan showed about 50 percent shrinkage of the two largest tumors in my lungs from the first CT scan in late November. There is continued improvement since January. The largest tumor, which was originally an egg-shaped mass, is now about 20 percent the size it was at Thanksgiving and is now an odd string-like shape. The original mass in the esophagus is still a thickening of the walls, but there is clearly a larger opening for food passage. I am certainly not cancer-free, but things are moving in the right direction. The doctor plans two to four more chemo infusions and then a cutback to a maintenance dose. He does not want me to be on the full treatment longer than six months. The maintenance treatment will include some intravenous meds, including one that I wear for forty-six hours as a pack and pump, but the strongest chemical—which creates the extreme cold sensitivity and some neuropathy—will be discontinued at least for a while. This may also allow me to get the hernia surgery I now need. In short, both improved health and ambiguity continue. All in all, it is a very good report.

* * * * * * *

The meaning issue I have been reflecting on these past two weeks is how one names one's struggle or journey with cancer. Why is it so often depicted in military terms—as a war, a battle, a fight, a conquering or a succumbing to the enemy? I have so often heard people say to me or others, "You are in the fight of—and for—your very life!" Is this image of warfare and battle really a healthy metaphor? Does this way of thinking actually lead to some dysfunctions in becoming healthy? As I was trying to think through this issue, I was intrigued to run across Walter Wangerin, Jr.'s comments (in *Letters from the Land of Cancer*), which seemed to be, at least, somewhat parallel to my own musings.

> [I refuse] to use the imagery of warfare when speaking of my cancer. I have never construed my cancer as my enemy... Please don't think I judge others who (thoughtfully) chose the image, for whom "fighting" may be a helpful attitude. On the other hand I am critical of the media... when without genuine forethought, they routinely declare, concerning a cancer death, that so-and-so has died "after a long battle with cancer."
>
> Why does it always have to be a "battle"? What?—are the folks fighting good cancer warriors if they win? (But what is winning?) Are they bad fighters—the unseated knights—if they lose? Often the media's sentimentalized characterization is that it was a "heroic" battle. But few other personal failures are praised as "heroic." Cancer isn't really an issue of defeat or victory. We are all going to die. (Wangerin, 2010: 160–161)

Wangerin raises some interesting issues, and I tend to agree with him, though my own struggle with this warlike language is a bit different. My body has not been invaded by a "foreign" or external virus or infection. Cancer is a case of one's own cells misbehaving. Failing to mature in a healthy way, all these cells want to do is procreate—to multiply and expand. Then they form an in-grown mass that tricks the body into thinking it is essential to the body—so the body creates artery and other connections to feed the mass. What does it mean to declare my own cells to be the "enemy"? What imagery and what attitudes of my being are influenced when I declare war or battle on my own cells? Is that constructive for my healing? Does that contribute to wholesome, healthy, vibrant, and harmonious physical and spiritual systems?

Some nations are more war-prone than others, and the United States is especially war-prone. The United States has been at war 201 of the 241 years since the colonies declared independence. Indeed, during the entire period from 1900 to the present, there were only six years when the United States has not been engaged in some sort of military action around the world (Mark Brandon, "War and Constitutional Order," *The Constitution in Wartime: Beyond Alarmism and Complacency*; Pedro Noguera and Robby, Cohen "Patriotism and Accountability: The Role of Education in the War on Terrorism," *Phi Delta Kappan*). We love war films, and we celebrate and laud the use of force to solve problems. Note that our history courses and our telling of U.S. history feature wars as the high points or turning points in our nation's development rather than highlighting human rights and peace movements as the defining feature of our country. It is no wonder that our language is so infused with warrior and battle metaphors.

Because he was trained in and wrote his dissertation on Boston Personalism, Martin Luther King, Jr. often cited a core principle of that philosophical tradition regarding social change: "The ends never justify the means, for the means are the end in process." This was why he insisted on *nonviolent* resistance. He believed that violence always led to a conflicted, violence-prone, coercive society rather than a healthy "beloved community." I think King was absolutely right, that the means of change and intended ends must be congruent. Not only is this true regarding social change (and is an insight many organizers for change fail to keep in mind), it is clearly true of teaching and learning. I learned long ago that some methodologies in the classroom (often including lecture if used extensively) are not conducive to deep learning or to critical thinking by students. Instructional methodologies need to be congruent with the anticipated and hoped-for learning outcomes. Clearly in a classroom, the means of instruction are the end in process.

Now I am rather inclined to think that this principle is true of most of life, and this is why personal integrity is so very important. Our means—the way we go about living our daily lives and the principles we embrace in everyday living—will shape the ultimate outcome: our character. If means and hoped-for outcomes must be congruent, that is unsettling when I think about declaring war on my own cells—using violent imagery directed to part of my own body. Somehow this metaphor of war or battle or aggression is discomforting; it does not resonate well. It seems like it cannot have an outcome of a harmonious, healthy, peaceful body and soul. Yet what other metaphor makes sense?

One core principle that Martin Luther King, Jr stressed regarding nonviolent resistance and realization of the beloved community is this: "Nonviolent resistance avoids not only external physical violence but also internal violence of the spirit. The nonviolent resister not only refuses to strike the opponent, but refuses to hate that opponent... This can only be done by projecting the ethic of love to the center of our lives" (King Stride, *Toward Freedom*, pp. 103–104). Wow! That is a tall order. Yet the core insight is that one must not let hatred, anger, or fear distort one's core being. Warrior imagery seems to foster aggression, fear, and demonization of part of one's body. Something deep in my bones tells me this is not healthy, is not a pathway to full health. At least it does not work for me.

An alternative metaphor—an alternative way of naming what I am going through—needs to express strength, purpose, and resilience, for those are essential parts of agency in a health crisis. It also needs to express some sort of transformation. In one sense, the imagery I use during meditation is a *melting* of the tumors—but that is not a real metaphor and does not fully express what I am going through. One idea—still a bit military in some sense—is to use an image from martial arts: the person in Tae Kwon Do or other such arts is trained to use the momentum and energy of the opponent against him or her—to sidestep and flip the energy a different way. Part of me likes that image, but it is not quite full enough to express the experience of dealing with a life-threatening ailment. Someone also has suggested to me that computer images may be useful: I am trying to *reboot* my life-forces. This is also an interesting idea, but I have not yet been able to unpack that image. I continue to be open to a healthy metaphor that depicts the struggle or "journey" of dealing with cancer and trying to heal (at least to the point of remission). If you have ideas for a nonviolent but strong metaphor, I would like to hear them. In the meantime, I think I have found one I like. This came to me during a meditative state while I was receiving healing touch energy treatment.

I have been working with a Dakota scholar to organize an Osher Lifelong Learning tour this summer on "Dakota Sacred Spaces and Places in the Twin Cites"—an experience I am very much looking forward to. One of the starting places is Indian Mounds Park in St. Paul, where there is a ravine that has been terribly abused and desecrated by whites. It had been a wetland ravine—a place of birthing and beginnings for the Dakota—but all the water had been drained, and it had become a dump fouled with pollutants and filled with refrigerators and other appliances that residents had tossed there. In recent years and with the help of some federal funds, the Dakota and others have been cleaning up this site. The trashed appliances have been removed, the water levels are coming back, and strategic native plants that either absorb chemicals or provide nutrients and renew the soil have been planted. All of this is done with a deep respect—a profound sacredness—for Mother Earth and for this particular site. It is hard work, but it is done with such love and positive energy. This seems to me to be a healthy metaphor for what I am hoping to accomplish within my own body—a *reclamation project*. I am trying to talk to my cells, to send positive energies to my esophagus, my lungs, and my lymph nodes and white blood cells. I do believe that love is more powerful and healthier than anger or aggression in converting and transforming any situation, including the reclamation of my body to health and wholeness.

In her sermon this week, Mayflower UCC Pastor Sarah Campbell stressed that gratitude begets generosity which begets gratitude which begets generosity. I think this is true, and gratitude is rooted in love, compassion, and commitment to the beloved community of justice, hope, and peace. There may be a better metaphor than *reclamation project*, but for now, this seems more congruent with a healthy body and thriving community, with generosity and gratitude, with positive energy and hope than the aggressive language of warfare, battles, and "heroic fighting." So if you use imagery in meditations and prayer, join with me in trying to name this effort as one of beloved reclamation of healthy cells—misbehaving cells that need to either dissolve or revert to healthy embryonic cells (which apparently is what does sometimes happen with redirected cancerous cells). I am trying to reclaim parts of my body that are malfunctioning and restore them to vitality. Moreover, if you identify another metaphor that expresses strength, purpose, resilience, and transformation and that conveys a means of healing that is congruent with love, community, and peaceful ends, I would love to hear your metaphor.

Clearly, my imagery recognizes parallels and connections between a healthy individual (micro) and healthy "beloved" community (macro). I do think they are profoundly linked, and they are both linked to a healthy Mother Earth. We are systems within systems within systems, not isolated atoms. That is why I see my own healing in larger social and environmental context. May we all embrace—and commit ourselves to—a healthy, beloved local community, national society, global village, and earth system.

Peace and love,
Keith

Gardening with Love and Communication

From Cindy Damm

Hi Keith,

Your search for a positive imagery is powerful in and of itself. I love to garden, and one of the things I've learned is that plants communicate not only with those of their own kind but also with those within a plant grouping or plant community. There are certain plants that choose to give up or allow themselves to weaken so that the remaining plants can be healthy. This is a phenomenon that appears to occur over and over with one or a few volunteering to attract the bad insects or forgo the water for the survival of the community. Oddly enough, I find it MUCH easier to pull weeds out if I ask them to let go literally, "Please let go, you can't grow here." It may seem strange, but if I forget to ask, I often find myself in a kind of tug-of-war to pull the plant's roots out. I recall that some hunters ask for permission before taking an animal's life. I wonder if it would be possible to imagine that these wayward cells would voluntarily give up, melt away, let go for the betterment of the community?

Love and appreciation,
Cindy

* * * * * *

Gardening

From Jane Legwold

Keith:

Your not liking the war-like/aggressive imagery rings true for me. My family has history of breast cancer that led me after genetic counseling to have prophylactic mastectomies back in 1995. Around that time, I went to a hypnosis conference that talked about the power of imagery and body-mind connection. The war imagery and battle language was aversive to me. But I am a gardener. I instead chose to use the imagery of my immune system being like a gardener, and I joined with it, discerning what were cancer cells and healthy cells, and weeded out the cancer/atypical cells as though they were weeds in my garden and discarded them with imagery outside of my body. My understanding is we all have atypical cells all the time, and just sometimes they take hold and proliferate. I felt peaceful with that imagery and in sync with my immune system. I had shared this with one of my colleagues, so when she was diagnosed with breast cancer and was doing her treatments, she used the imagery of the white-scarfed women in maybe Monet's paintings—lovely imagery—and expanded beyond herself to a whole team of women weeding the fields. Again, thanks for your thought-provoking writing that you are sharing with us. You are such a gift to us all with your wise reflections.

Jane

* * * * * *

Plants...

From Pam Larson

I'd never given much thought to the fact that military terms are used to "fight" cancer. Interesting! I like what Wangerin says. In my dad's obituary, we used "brief struggle with cancer," and I see "battle" used often in obituaries. I think for Dad's obituary, it was more to let people know that he didn't suffer for years with cancer—as well as letting people know what took his life—and using "brief bout with cancer" seemed to minimize his end. Good food for thought there.

I really like your imagery of being a reclamation project! You need a native plant to visualize as something you would plant in your reclamation project, one that will neutralize the cancer. Nobel Prize winner Dr. Otto Warburg, discovered that cancer cells could not exist in the presence of abundant oxygen Herb Robert has a unique ability to make more oxygen available to the cells, which means the body has the opportunity to fight disease more effectively.

I hope that resonates with you, Keith. Plants are truly miraculous, especially the plants that can absorb and "de-fuse" toxins. Even non-native house plants can absorb formaldehyde, benzene, toluene, etc. Incredible. Herb Robert is such a beautiful and delicate-looking plant, but apparently it's a powerful beauty!

10

Awkward!—What to Say (or Not Say) to Friends with a Life-threatening Disease

April 17, 2017

Family, friends,

My Mayo Clinic infusion room this time has a window, and it is a gorgeous blue-sky day. My writing gives me some sense of purpose in sitting here for four hours, so I hope I have something useful to communicate. My blood platelets number is slightly below the desired levels, but all immunity indicators are solid. I had a bit more neuropathy in my fingers and toes this past two-week period, but after today, I will have only two more infusions with the strongest of the medications (oxaliplatin). I did not see a doctor this time, so there is not much more to report. I am incredibly fortunate because I have no pain at all, and my energy levels are really quite good. I simply do not feel ill. My main negative is that since September, when I became more acutely aware that something was amiss, I have lost almost thirty pounds. I continue to use multiple strategies in this reclamation/restoration project: strong attention to diet; roughly thirty minutes of meditation (most days); seventy-five minutes of "healing touch" ministry every other week; Qi-ssage acupressure massage on the alternate week; and continual awareness and deep gratitude for the prayers, daily lit candles, meditative energy transference, and other supportive actions that people all across this country have taken on my behalf. Your presence in my life is palpable.

* * * * * * *

One issue I have been reflecting on in the last two weeks is those awkward moments when someone says something that is quite unhelpful or just profoundly awkward. The awkward statement may well occur because the person is not effectively taking the role of the ill individual before speaking, but I think a situation often becomes uncomfortable because so many people feel awkward around one who is not well or who is immediately challenged by death. We want to say something, but what we say is sometimes odd at best. Walter Wagerin says this about many exchanges he experienced in the depths of his "reclamation project" with cancer:

> Already now, the day before my first chemothera-peutic session, people who know of my cancer have repeated well-meant formulas in such a way as to indicate a distance between themselves and me.
>
> Well, what can you say to someone with a killing disease? Especially when you are not practiced at the conversation—and when you yourself feel the difference, as if the afflicted one has been removed from the common life and a kind of cellophane wraps him away? (Wagerin, *Letters from the Land of Cancer*, p. 32)

Walter Wagerin—as well as other narrators I have read—note that a person with a life-threatening disease experiences distancing and isolation, as if she or he is no longer fully part of the community. He is treated as though he already has a foot in the casket or the urn, and the consequence (quite unintended) can be to make the ill person feel diminished. I must say that I have only experienced this myself once or twice, but I understand the feeling. Some people have seemed to expect me to be vulnerable and frail, treating me with kid gloves, though I am in no pain at all and my energy levels are good. In any case, I have been intrigued by the awkwardness that does sometimes arise and have wondered about its source and its meaning.

Because of this distancing, sociological studies by scholars like Kathy Charmaz have demonstrated that many ill people try to hide their illness, or at least the severity of it. That in itself is a strain—one more added to the ambiguity and perhaps fears or confusion at the plethora of decisions to be made. So how do we engage with people in a way that is not strained or stressful? I hesitate to wade into these waters, for I do not have extensive data for making a generalization nor am I highly familiar with the counseling literature in this area. I am also aware that each individual constructs or makes meaning out of interactions in ways that reflect his or her own personal history, and not all will respond the way I do. Things I find awkward or vacuous may not be so for others. However, I will be foolishly bold by entering this discussion and hope some of you have better advice than my musings.

It is interesting how one immediately picks up on deep sympathy from people, and yet… and yet. Sympathy somehow feels uncomfortable, and I think two issues are in play. Sympathy can feel like one is already on the way down the tubes, and people are waving goodbye. I am very much still in survival mode. As I wrote in the last chronicle, the warlike language of battles or fighting does not resonate well with me. However, I am involved in the hard work of a reclamation (or restoration) project and am not really looking for "sympathy." What is more helpful than sympathy is *moral support*. (I do get a lot of that too.)

The second problem with sympathy is it communicates that the person is weak, vulnerable, or in some sense ineffectual. Sympathy can sometimes be experienced as the strong offering compensation to the weaker person. There are, indeed, clear rules for when to be sympathetic and how to express it, and it often involves higher prestige persons commiserating with an underling. When a subordinate communicates sympathy to a person higher in the social system, it must be done very carefully, if at all. These patterns were found in research by Candace Clark ("Sympathy, Biography, and Sympathy Margin,"

American Journal of Sociology). (In case you are interested, I will include at the end of this essay a listing of the key "social rules for sympathy" that Clark identified.) While the person expressing sympathy may not perceive it as an expression that is any way a one-up expression, according to some scholars who have studied this type of interaction, it is not uncommon for it to be perceived this way. This power or status perception may be why sociologist Kathy Charmaz (*Good Days, Bad Days: The Self in Chronic Illness*) found that so many people hide their illness, or at least its severity. Being ill may make one immediately appear less competent and less vital. It is valuable to, at least, know that severe illness means your friend, acquaintance, or family member is not only dealing with the emotional strain of coping with lowered energy and perhaps pain but is also very possibly experiencing significant social marginalization at the same time. So my suggestion is to be supportive, which is different from being sympathetic. Say you are saddened if that is true, but follow it with support.

One of the most important things, I think, in interacting with folks struggling with a life-threatening disease is this: *no platitudes or shibboleths, please.* There is no doubt that people (including me) offer these with good intentions and because they feel so awkward that they don't know what else to say. Here are some examples:

- "Everything happens for a reason." Awk! What? This is obviously false, but more importantly, it communicates to the ill person that she/he somehow deserved this or is supposed to take a moral lesson from this health calamity. Many things in life are random; as my biologist friend, Dennis McDonald, likes to say, somewhat tongue in cheek, "Life is what actually happens to you while you are planning your life." Now we can *choose* to seek meaning and an opportunity for personal growth in any situation, but those paths are based on personal agency in finding how one might learn and grow from the adversity. That is part of the challenge for Judy and me—to create meaning and seek opportunities for growth from this unwelcome twist in the road. The notion that everything happens for a reason assumes the meaning is both inherent in the events themselves and it obscure. It is a horrible platitude that just makes the person feel worse. It is clearly *not supportive.*

- "God never gives you more than you can handle." Again, this is so obviously false that it is mean-spirited to say it. It is also terrible theology! Many people are faced with more than they can handle: think of parents unable to protect their children in the Nazi concentration camps or mothers trying to keep their babies and young children alive in famine-stricken refugee camps. Every day there are people in our country whose coping mechanisms have been overwhelmed, and they commit suicide. It is our God-given responsibility to stop tragedies, but God will not solve the issue without human intervention and engagement. Let's not get into the nasty business of blaming God for malady and mayhem we experience; it can only generate resentment toward God. Let us recognize this for what it is—a shibboleth (a misleading saying or half-truth, at best, that is propagated in a particular ethnic, faith, ideological, or political community). It is more damaging than helpful, even though it is said with good intentions.

- "You are going to be okay. I just know it." Of course, you do *not* know it, and the person hearing it knows it is a vacuous platitude. It feels insincere, and although most of us hearing such a comment know that you are just feeling awkward and want to say something, it is frankly not reassuring. Now if you know this person well and know her to be a deeply resourceful person—a person of grit and grace and gratitude, then say that! Notice how different this sounds: "I have never really said this to you before, but I have always seen you as a person of such courage and positive energy. It gives me hope that if anyone can master this, you can. I am pulling for you and would be honored to be supportive in any way I can."

- My friend, Chris Wilcox, who is currently dealing with a recurrence of cancer after more than a decade of clean bills of health, says one of the most awkward things people say is "What's your prognosis?" She writes, "I want to say, 'What's *your* prognosis?' We are not immortal; no one knows what will happen around the bend." I probably was among the first to ask Chris if she was given a prognosis when she went through her first successful cancer reclamation/restoration. I now see what she means. For one thing, I have explicitly not asked my doctor what my "prognosis" is since I do not want it to become a reverse placebo effect—where I come to expect to live only that long. Further, many people are not ready to self-disclose details—in part because it takes them further out of the mainstream and makes them seem like one foot is in the grave. Asking specific questions about ailments or prognosis may feel intrusive. So find ways to open the door without being probing.

- "Oh, my mom had it twice, and she beat it." It may be helpful to hear that others have been successful in restoration of their bodies to health—it can signal hope—but it is not supportive when one makes it sound like a walk in the park. Tone can be a key in being supportive.
- Silence or avoidance. Some people never mention the illness, though they know about it. The illness is the elephant in the room, and pretending it is not there can make some people feel invisible. Of course, the illness must not be the sole topic of conversation. The illness is neither the defining characteristic of the person nor the only subject of interest to him. Talk about common interests (politics, sports, common concerns of the community), but be aware that pretending there is no elephant at all is not experienced as support. The key is to be honest, willing to listen, supportive, and interested in the person as a whole person, not just a diseased one.

In pointing out clumsy and hurtful things that people may say to someone who is vulnerable and very ill, perhaps the biggest mistake one can make is to become so afraid of misspeaking that one simply withdraws. Sometimes we have to move forward with our words of support but always scrutinizing our own actions or words for unintended consequences. If one sincerely apologizes for clumsy, insensitive comments, most people will understand and forgive the gaff. Most people will focus on the good intentions rather than the words themselves. I do hope these cautions do not cause further intimidation and reticence to engage someone with cancer. I write of these "word wounds" only so people can be more aware that many of our culture's tired expressions and clichés are thoughtless and painful to hear from the other side of the bed stand. My purpose is to examine—using a sociological lens—what is going on in these exchanges.

So how do I make sense of what is happening in these awkward moments? Within microsociology, there is a specialty area in the sociology of emotions that analyzes "emotional labor." It has focused largely on study of people whose job is to manage the feelings of other people (counselors are an obvious example). One brilliant study by Arlie Russell Hochschild (*The Managed Heart: Commercialization of Human Feeling*) focused on the work of flight attendants and how they had to manage or control their own feelings in order to keep the emotions of travelers on an even keel. For flight attendants, sometimes on-the-job management of their own feelings comes at a cost to their private lives since they had been repressing anger or frustration or other feelings they could not express. Repression is exhausting, and the repressed feelings often explode in another context. This raises interesting questions about "the commercialization of emotions"—when one is *paid to manage emotions*. It is a fascinating field of study.

One of the most interesting studies in this subfield is on how some people are forced to engage in emotional labor because others respond to them as oddities or are very obviously uncomfortable around them. The most telling study to me was research by Spencer Cahill and Robin Eggleston on how much energy it takes for wheelchair users to put able-bodied people at ease around them ("Wheelchair Users' Interpersonal Management of Emotions," *Social Psychology Quarterly*). They must learn strategies such as humor and assertiveness in defining the situation so that TABs (the temporarily able-bodied) are comfortable. It can be exhausting to have to put other people at ease. I think that one thing many people with a life-threatening ailment must do is to engage in emotional labor, and that means learning strategies for putting other people at ease. So you might be aware in interacting with seriously ill people that they may carry an extra burden of needing to put you and others around you at ease in order to "normalize" the interaction and reduce strain. They may be feeling an obligation to perform emotional labor (though they may not be familiar with the term itself). The most compassionate and supportive thing you can do is to be a genuine friend and not put the person in the position of both having to cope with both her own confused and convoluted emotions about the illness and to perform emotional labor to help you manage your emotions.

I do not think there is any formula for what to say. Genuineness, honesty, and support are always at the core of constructive interactions in cases like this. Here are a few examples of entries into genuine conversations:

- You might simply let the person know that they are in your thoughts, your heart, your prayers. Sometimes it is appropriate and genuine to say that you will be thinking of (praying for) that person daily, or lighting a candle each day as a reminder of his struggle, or sending positive energy through meditative imagery. This is simple but *supportive.*

- You might want to ask about what kind of prayer or meditation is desired. Some people may want prayers for healing. Others may not think that is possible at this stage but want to be pain-free, or want to have energy to finish a project, or want prayers for their children or partner. Asking if there are specific requests for prayer/meditation may open doors for the person to talk and to disclose concerns—but the ill person is entirely in control of the disclosure.

- You might ask if there are any tangible ways you can be supportive—meals, raking a yard, snow removal, something else that would be beneficial.

- It may be appropriate to express appreciation for what that person has meant to you, not in a morbid way, but with appreciation and with empathy with the person's struggles. This might be done in writing or in person but is an affirmation of the person's gifts, her contributions to one's own life, her inspiration (if that is the case). This needs to be expressed as a method of passing along energy-enhancing positivity, which you have received from that person on previous occasions.

- I realize that some people (including those who are ill) are contact avoidant, but I find that some of the most eloquent statements of support are hugs. Several people at our church say little (or maybe say something simple like, "Thinking of you daily and sending positive energy your way") but offer a warm embrace. It expresses deep support.

- Perhaps saying something like this would be an option: "I can't possibly fully enter into or understand what you are going through, but I would be most willing to listen if you want to talk out loud about the experience or just need to vent. I do not want you to go through this alone, and I am willing to be there." Then call the person a few days later, asking if he or she would like to meet at a coffee shop. Also let the ill friend know that if he/she already has more than enough support or is just not at a point where to be ready to share, that it is fine to be straight about that. You will not be offended. Make it clear that you offer support but do not want to be intrusive if the person just needs space. Finally, always remember that your first job is simply to *listen* and be supportive. Your own thoughts are not what the person needs as much as your *presence*.

As I write this, I am reminded of a self-deprecating but poignant story told by the eminent American theologian, Reinhold Niebuhr, in *Leaves from the Notebook of a Tamed Cynic*. Niebuhr was a young, very green pastor, fresh out of seminary and only a week or two into his first position as the minister of a local church. Someone important in the congregation (we'll call him Owen Jones) had died, and he was called immediately to do pastoral care. He did not have a clue what to do or say, but he showed up at the home of the deceased and was invited in by the Jones family. He was pretty speechless, not wanting to spout meaningless platitudes, so he just sat in the living room and listened. He would ask an occasional question but was embarrassed by his own ineptitude as a spiritual support and counselor. After sitting on the couch—rather like a bump on a log—for several hours, he excused himself and went home to work on his Sunday sermon. That was difficult to concentrate on since he was feeling utterly incompetent as a pastor. Several weeks later, he heard from a member of the congregation that the community was delighted with his leadership and that he had a reputation for being especially skilled in comforting those who are grieving. The Jones family had reported to many people that Rev. Niebuhr was just exceptional as a support to them. Sometimes silent listening is golden!

I love the story because it illustrates how simple support can often be. Interacting with people who are ill or with people who are bereaved need not be awkward and result in awkward platitudes. It is better to keep silent while being *profoundly present* to the person. As Rachel Naomi Remen, M.D. writes in *Kitchen Table Wisdom: Stories that Heal*, "Perhaps the most important thing we ever give to each other is our attention... A loving silence often has more power to heal and to connect than the most well-intentioned words." Simply be a friend—not a friend of a sick person but a friend. If this is the approach, you are less likely to feel awkward and to make less than helpful comments. You are less likely to put the ill person in the position of doing emotional labor to manage your feelings of awkwardness.

You may have more insight into ways to be supportive and to reduce awkwardness than those strategies I suggest here, and I would love to hear your ideas. I will close with one story about grief itself and how to be supportive since I think it is relevant to and consistent with these musings.

When my father died and we really were in grief, there were many cards that came to the house, some of them with odd platitudes that rang inauthentic or untrue. We focused on the intent to comfort rather than the messages themselves. There was one message, however, a message I have used many times since to send to those deeply bereaved, that spoke profoundly to me and to Judy. It was the words of that great theologian, mystic, university Chaplain (and a mentor to Martin Luther King, Jr. at Boston University), Howard Thurman. In many ways, it communicates the same tone and invitation to dialogue that I have been suggesting be employed in interactions with the seriously ill—quiet, unassuming support. I will end with his thoughtful words.

For a Time of Sorrow
Howard Thurman

I share with you the agony of your grief,
    The anguish of your heart finds echo in my own.
    I know I cannot enter all you feel
    Nor bear with you the burden of your pain;

I can but offer what my love does give:
    The strength of caring,
    The warmth of one who seeks to understand
    The silent storm-swept barrenness of so great a
loss.

This I do in quiet ways,
    That on your lonely path
    You may not walk alone.

Sociologists insist that even human emotions are "socially patterned"— that is, emotions are not simply spontaneous feelings. They change according to culture, according to membership in different groups within a society, and according to one's social status within a given society. This principle applies to both how we express emotions and to what we feel. Much of this analysis focuses on the role of reciprocity and the way we create sympathy "accounts" that can be used—or abused—by breaking social rules of when and how to express sympathy.

Social Rules Governing the Sympathy Responses in the U.S.

Candace Clark

1. *Do not make false or needless claims to sympathy.* It will offend people and reduce your sympathy account, so it is empty when you really do need some support.
2. *Do not claim too much sympathy.* Again, overdrawing on sympathy will create an overdrawn account.

3. *Do not accept sympathy too readily.* Some people seem too eager for sympathy, and it offends and reduces one's credibility for real sympathy when needed.

4. *Do claim* <u>*some*</u> *sympathy when it is offered, or you will not have any when you need it.* Clark writes: "The self-reliant—who remain independent and do not develop sympathy "credit ratings" by borrowing and repaying—may not have sympathy accounts in time of need."

5. *Reciprocate to others for the gift of sympathy and be sensitive to differences in social status or standing within the social group in determining how you respond.*

    a) Payment of sympathy does not have to return to the original donor, but failure to be sympathetic to others if you have received sympathy may cause ill feelings toward you.

    b) Payment of sympathy may be expressed simply in gratitude to the other.

    c) Gifts of sympathy from persons who are of higher status (e.g. "the Boss") are of greater value than other sympathy. Sympathy is often from a more powerful or prestigious member of the social group to someone of lesser status, as it is a subtle statement of dominance in who "owes" whom. Receiving sympathy puts one in a position of "owing" or being *obligated* to the other, and those in power *often* (there are exceptions) do not appreciate being put in that position. Therefore, the *payment of gratitude* to a superior may need to be in the form of *deference.*

(Candace Clark "Sympathy, Biography, and Sympathy Margin," *American Journal of Sociology*)

Peace and love,
Keith

11

The Challenge of Cancer to a Coherent and Healthy Self

May 1, 2017

Family, friends,

It is infusion day in room 29 of the Mayo Clinic's Gonda Building, tenth floor. I muse and reflect; thus, I write. Most of my immunity numbers are in the low normal range. I only have two more infusions with this oxaliplatin chemo, and the doctor today cut the dosage for the last two treatments to 50 percent of the original dose. This is partially due to the neuropathy I have been experiencing in my hands, which they do not want to become permanent. At the outset of the treatment, the doctor had said that radiation was off the table because this is stage 4 cancer, and it is not localized. However, the tumors in my lungs have shrunk very substantially, as has the swelling in my lymph glands. It appears that the mass in my esophagus is harder to impact because of the type of tissue and because the "nutrients" available to the malignancy are different. So there is now some discussion by my oncology team that a round of radiation (for perhaps five weeks) might be needed and effective. I would likely be off chemo for that period, and that might be a time when I could also have the hernia surgery that I need done. So on my next trip to Mayo, I will likely be meeting with a radiation oncologist and a surgeon. My energy remains very good, my spirits are positive, and I have no pain.

At the urging of many of you, my readers, I have taken a few steps toward possible publication of these reflections as a book. I sent off a cover letter and the first nine entries to the acquisitions editor (I did not have a name) of two publishing houses that have published a number of books on cancer or mortality issues, including cancer journals or letters. I have yet to hear anything after nearly a month, and it may well be that I have to first find an agent to help get a foot in the door.

I have published more than twenty books, including revised editions (that fact alone would likely put both my high school and college English teachers in shock), but those were all academic books (textbooks or monographs for other professors). So I am a novice at figuring out how to publish with a large commercial house. Our son, Kent, a writer, tells me I need to create a substantial prospectus that includes comparisons with similar works in the genre and provides marketing information to convince them they will make a healthy profit. College comrade and retired English Professor Joel Wingard also had some useful advice. So it seems I have to do writing that I do not really want to do in order to publish the kind of reflective writing that is stimulating, and even therapeutic, to me. I doubt that my current title—at least, as the primary title—would draw much interest from browsing bookstore folks, so I am contemplating another option: *Making Meaning in the Midst of Malignancy*. (Yes, I know—I am a *hopeless* alliterator.) In any case, if you happen to know how to open the door or have the key to a commercial publishing house editor, I'd be interested.

* * * * * * *

I write this essay on meaning-making regarding cancer and selfhood with some trepidation, for I will be stepping into some theory that may be a bit dense at points. I will try to illustrate to flesh out the concepts. Regardless, the issue is one that has existential importance for me as I reflect on my experience and read about others. Many people find that their sense of self takes a serious hit with chronic illness, and a result is hurt, embitterment, and even depression. Is there an alternative path for fragile selfhood in the midst of severe health affliction?

In my previous entry on what to say (or not say) to someone with cancer, I touched on how illness creates vulnerabilities and sometimes social isolation or marginalization. The underlying issue is how illness impacts the sense of self in sometimes profound ways. Thus far, I have remained pretty healthy and energetic, and I have experienced only bits of this personally, but I have been reading about the social psychology of illness and musing on why it is important for ill people and those who care about them to understand the potential impact of illness on sense of self. In order for this discussion to make sense, I need to delve into some sociological ideas about the self and its emergence.

Words are pretty amazing, among other things, allowing us to create feelings in one another. My words alone might stimulate emotions in you: fear, sympathetic pain, direct pain (informing you of death of a family member that occurred in another location), nervousness, exhilaration, or depression. One powerful role of words is names—through which we can symbolically objectify self and others. This "objectification" allows us to discuss someone who is not present amongst us. I say the name Judy Roberts, and we both have a face, a personality, an image in our minds of the same person. We can talk about her (either in a complementary way or we could be catty and "gossip" about her—heaven forbid!) because we both think of interactions with this one person. Yet this very capacity to name also allows me to objectify myself. It allows me to talk about myself in third person, *and* it allows me to talk *to* myself as I consider how I should broach a sensitive topic in conversation with someone. A friend of mine once made the humorous comment, "Sometimes I get on my own nerves." That indicates reflection on self, and even self-criticism, as if it were another person being discussed. This requires role-taking or perspective-taking ability.

Perspective-taking allows me to control my behavior. It permits me to reflect on my actions or my persona, to critique my conduct, and thereby to modify my actions. Through role-taking and anticipation of negative consequences, I can avoid certain behaviors. I can also learn from the mistakes of others rather than having to make the mistake myself and experience the consequences—all because of language and role-taking. It is pretty marvelous—a gift we often take for granted. Without a symbol for "self"—one's name—this could not happen.

In microsociology, George Herbert Mead framed this role—taking process as the interaction of the *I* and the *me*. The *I* is the *subjective* experience of the actor, while the *me* refers to the objectification process of the reflector. The individual begins to act (perhaps to say something), and the *me* role-takes and places the self as an object. The person mentally steps outside of herself and looks back, noticing that a current behavior or a planned action would be condemned by herself and her associates if it were done by another member of the community. The *I* then changes course and reconsiders. One might, for example, examine how to word something by taking the point of view of one's audience. (Hmmm. Better not use that term since someone in the room is from that ethnic group and might find "Native American" problematic and prefer "first nations.")

The *I* is spontaneous and often impulsive ("Did I really do that?" "I can't believe I actually said that!"). The *Me* allows a corrective based on role-taking. In short, one is imagining that one is seeing though the eyes of associates, friends, or a "generalized other." The *Me* is the dimension of self that allows us to talk *to* ourselves and *about* ourselves in third person and to anticipate perceptions and reactions of others. Before I teach a class of traditional college students, I have to stop and think about what examples will be interesting and meaningful to eighteen-to-twenty-two-year-olds rather than people my own age. I have to role-take with the anticipated audience.

Sometimes there is tension between the *I* and the *me*; the *I* wants to act and refuses to be corrected. If I am angry at that moment, I may just not give a damn about consequences. Anger may prevent me from self-control; it overrules my "better judgment." (I may later wish I had listened to the *me* that was trying to tell me, "Stop!") In Mead's formulation then, *self is the interaction between one's I and one's me."* A healthy person must have both at work, and sense of self needs to be based on multiple dimensions of belonging and conduct.

Some fascinating studies have shown that people who receive inordinate acclamation and attention for one portion of the self—such as extraordinary athletic ability that brings glory or exceptional physical beauty find that others respond to them almost entirely on the basis of that trait or skill (Patricia Adler and Peter Adler "The Gloried Self," *Social Psychology Quarterly*). Persons who experience this lopsided authentication and praise often develop a truncated or "flat" sense of self that does not serve well over time. It may even keep one locked in glory past. It undermines development of a multidimensional sense of identity. Receiving disproportionate attention or glory for one dimension of self is dangerous to healthy selfhood.

The heart of the process of healthy self-evolution then is role-taking, a skill that is absolutely essential to much that is important in life: emergence of the self; self-reflection; all forms of human cooperation; learning from the past; planning for the future; controlling, directing, or leading others; love; all forms of critical thinking/analysis; and all forms of ethical reflection. This is why I have argued through most of my career that expansion of perspective-taking should be the single most important objective for all sociology instruction: clearly one cannot do sociology without expanded perspective-taking to see things from a different place on the social landscape.

The *self* then is a product of social interaction. John Hewitt (*Self and Society*, eighth edition) writes, "There is no self at birth, only an organism capable of acquiring selfhood. The neonate does not yet have language, and so lacks the developed symbolic capacity for self-designation. Hence, the infant neither acts toward itself as an object, nor is its behavior regulated by a dialogue between *I* and *me*" (p. 79). Cooley actually called this a "looking glass self," for the self is what is reflected back to us in the mirror provided by others. Moreover, cultivation and remolding *of the self* is (or should be) a lifelong developmental process as we learn to see things through new lenses and the perspectives of those very unlike ourselves.

The glitch is that cancer or another life-threatening ailment can throw a wrench into this reflection process in ways I had not previously understood. As I wrote in my previous meaning-making essay, having a major illness can make one feel vulnerable—even fragile—and can cause others to question one's competency (professionally or personally). This is why disclosure versus transparency is such a hard choice for many people. To disclose is to risk being pitied, marginalized, or diminished as less than whole. So while having a life-threatening disease is itself an emotional drag, as people are weakened in really intense parts of their journey, their very sense of self may be impacted. As Kathy Charmaz writes in *Good Days and Bad Days: The Self in Chronic Illness and Time*, "Having a chronic illness means more than learning to live with it. It means struggling to maintain control over the defining images of self and over one's life" (Charmaz, p. 5). She expands this:

> The monitoring *me* defines the *I*'s behaviors, feelings, impulses, and sensations. It evaluates them and plans action to meet defined needs. Here, an ill person takes his or her physical self as an object, appraises it, and compares it with past selves, with perceived health status of others, [and] with ideals of physical or mental well-being." (p. 71).

When one is ill with an ailment that may never be overcome, the *me* sees a different person than a month or a year before. I have always been vigorous and had robust health, and my energy and strength have been remarkably hearty, but that is not entirely what my *me* sees nowadays. Other things that have been a core part of my reflected self are also in some jeopardy. I have always just loved teaching—the interaction, the process of working with things of the mind, the reflected image of self that I receive from my students. Teaching gives me an affirmation as a knowledgeable and skilled teacher and a competent human being. I am continuing to teach in the OLLI (Osher Lifelong Learning Institute) program with seniors, and I thrive on that. Yet I wonder if my energies were too low to conduct ninety-minute classes, what would my *me* see?

Even the aging process tends to undermine healthy self since our culture is so youth-oriented. In his new documentary, *The New Old*, David Carey examines the negative media messages of old people as being less than competent. Rather than elders being seen as uniquely qualified sources of wisdom that the society urgently needs, elders are depicted as out-of-date, technologically inept, and "post-adult." Illness escalates the process of demeaning a person. Certainly, having a terminal illness is the ultimate form of being a "lame duck." As one's life-force and capabilities do wane with disease, a positive sense of self and identity is increasingly difficult. Perhaps this is why so many people in later years of life become bitter, cynical, and filled with negative energy. If I want to avoid this negativity and bitterness, what do I do to sustain a positive sense of self? I know people—like Dana Blanck (one of our beloved church's musicians) who died from cancer this past weekend—whose entire persona radiated something healthy and wholesome and affirming, so it is very possible to sustain positivity.

In addition to a declining reflected self, a debilitating illness has a way of taking over life plans and priorities. Again, Charmaz's study of people coping with illness is instructive: "Although illness orders life, it does not entirely define or fill it… [But] when life becomes founded on illness… people must reconstruct their lives. The requirements of illness and health come first" (Charmaz, p.76). So even my ability to maintain priorities and make choices based on core values—essential in feeling agency—may be under threat.

Of course, part of one's sense of self is also connecting to the past—to the things one has tried to affirm in one's life and to the ways one has felt competent. However, a health crisis creates disruption, even in one's sense of time and continuity. Charmaz found that "in crises, a radically changed present separates one from the past. Like a guillotine, the crisis severs the present from the past and shatters the future. Hence, ill people feel severed and swept away from their pasts into an uncontrollable present and future" (p. 33). I have not experienced that at this point, but I can understand it—can hear it resonate in a deep sense that I did not comprehend prior to my current experience of trying to reclaim my health. She also says that people in more intense states of illness talk a good deal about "good days" and "bad days."

> Evaluations of days are fundamentally intertwined with evaluations of self. Ill people measure the quality of the day against the self they recognize, acknowledge, and wish to be. Thus, they judge whether the day is consistent with the self they wish to affirm and resend to others… Bad days elicit anger and frustration because they negate being one's preferred self. (Charmaz pp. 50, 52).

So illness and the social processes surrounding illness can "negate being one's preferred self." That seems to me to be the heart of the matter and the core of my musings for today. It may be why so many people have such strong emotional reactions, including depression.

How do I keep a negation of preferred self from happening? I have long affirmed Mead's concept of the self being the interaction between the *I* and the *me*. Still, this dance with cancer has caused me to question whether this framing is a bit too transient and perhaps delimiting. The me is seeing things through the eyes of others—role-taking and looking back at an objectified or third-person self. At this point in my life, I feel that what I need is an even broader or deeper perspective in which I compare myself to an ideal self—my notion of my best self as I understand that in my most reflective moments.

In those most insightful reflective moments, I understand myself as a responsible self and participant in a global community that is "sacred" in its core. What am I called to be—now, today—in that context? So instead of critiquing self in light of what others might say (the *me* cautioning the *I* that I am about to annoy someone), I am sensing that I need to be critiquing self in light of an *ideal self* or what we might even call a *transcendent self.* This calls for me personally to seek ways to pursue justice and compassion in whatever ways I can, at both the macro level of society and at the most micro level of social interaction in everyday life. This is the kind of person I would like to be, but I know that I often fall short. Others may have different notions of "best self" against which they can measure who they are. This suggested alternative moves me from a descriptive/analytical approach to a normative notion of selfhood. In this way, perhaps I can sustain a positive presence and defy bitterness, for I would not be subject to the tyranny of other's judgments about my current persona. Charmaz concludes, "Illness does not necessarily fill or flood the self, even though it may fill and flood experience... Transcendence implies reevaluation and renewal. Achieving transcendence requires making choices and taking action (*Good Days, Bad Days: The Self in Chronic Illness*, p. 258).

Although I have been unable to trace the original source, endocrinologist and philosopher Deepak Chopra is widely quoted as saying, "Every cell in your body is eavesdropping on your thoughts (quoted by Patrick Quillin in Beating Cancer with Nutrition, p. 105). (Note: I have learned since originally writing this that a very similar statement—that "our cells are listening to our thoughts"—came from Nobel prize-winning molecular biologist Elizabeth Blackburn and psychologist Elissa Epel in *The Telomere Effect: A Revolutionary Approach to Living Younger,*

Healthier, Longer.) If there is even a kernel of truth to this, then ridding ourselves of negativity and bitterness is crucial to an anticancer life.

I hope what I have written here makes sense and is not just nerdy ruminations of a pontificating professor. What I am trying to suggest is an alternative reference point for my *me* to provide feedback to my *I*. (Hmmm. I also seem to be inventing new grammar!) I am hoping this is a more constructive and less vulnerable perspective on self in society. It seems to me I can seek to be my best self despite current setbacks in my physical condition. I risk writing this abstract essay because I hope it might provide insights for those caretakers and friends who are well into the emotional roller coaster that very ill people experience (including depression and diminution of self-esteem). You can help others, perhaps, in their struggles with debilitating illness or disability by helping them make autonomous choices—for agency promotes and nurtures self-respect.

I hope that for those who are ill, these musings can provide an alternative path for reflecting on self—one that is less susceptible to the less-than-positive images one experiences from companions or the media. If it is you who faces that debilitation, perhaps focusing on the self you want to be—your best self—and concentrating on the legacy you wish to leave will help you rise above the petty things that can undermine positive selfhood and identity. Even if one feels weak and enervated, one can strive to be humane and a person of integrity. Please know that I affirm your efforts to do so; you and I will press on together in a countercultural and perhaps counterintuitive struggle to rise above pessimism and negativity. I hope you can find or create some plausibility structures (Chronicle 4) that sustain you in that journey.

Peace and love,
Keith

12

Planning for the Future When "Planning the Future" Feels like an Oxymoron

May 15, 2017

Family, friends,

While awaiting admission at the Mayo Clinic's chemo infusion waiting room, I overheard a conversation by three men who were sharing stories about their cancer situations. One man, who actually looked quite good, was thankful that he will survive to see his son's wedding next week. He will have witnessed the marriages of all three of his children but lamented the fact that he would never know any of his grandchildren. He has esophageal cancer and was given a twenty-month prognosis some sixteen months ago. He commented, "We make no plans at all for the future because there really is no future for me." I found the comment interesting since "the future" was what I was intending to write about today.

My blood counts are all quite strong today, and I really do feel great. Mayo Clinic is an amazing medical center in the allopathic tradition, but I must admit I have been appalled by the advice I have been getting from the nutrition folks at various allopathic cancer centers. So this past week, I started with a naturopath that our son, Kent, likes a lot. He has many suggestions for nutrition and gaining weight back that do not involve sugar. Forty percent of chemo-related deaths are due to malnutrition, so I am taking the weight loss seriously. The naturopath, Dr. Litchy, confirmed that within his discipline, chemo was the right way to go for the type and stage of cancer I have, and he agreed that the next step may need to be a round of radiation. Having said that, he has specific dietary suggestions that he has found will mitigate the side effects of radiation.

My naturopathy doctor wants me to try acupuncture and also strongly recommended hyperthermal therapy. I had been reading about hyperthermal treatments from a number of sources. It seems that something about cancer cells makes them vulnerable to heat, so the idea is that through hot tubs, extremely hot showers, or (best of all) saunas, one gets the body above 107 degrees, and then cancer cells start dying off. Daughter Elise (and husband Brett) have a sauna, so with our son, Justin, visiting again from Alaska, I did a half hour at about 180 degrees in the sauna. I was totally exhausted afterwards and napped for two hours, but I must say that I felt *terrific*. I had less "chest pressure" in the sternum area than I had had for months. I may well decide to cook myself at least once a week.

After my early morning chemo treatment today (beginning at six fifteen), I will meet with a radiology oncologist. With my tumor so close to the heart, the question of collateral damage is one I will be probing.

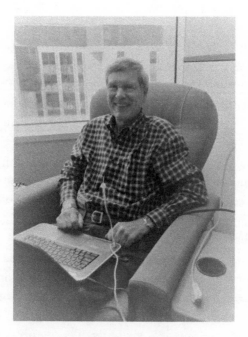

* * * * * * *

Later Update: I did meet with the radiology oncologist after the infusion. One form of radiation treatment is highly focused—more laser-like—and, therefore, has less collateral damage to other organs. It is called proton radiation therapy. The Mayo Clinic is the only cancer center in Minnesota that has this newest technology, so it would mean daily trips to Rochester, Minnesota, for five and a half weeks (twenty-eight treatments). Often in palliative therapy, they do three weeks, but the radiation oncologist and my primary oncologist (Dr. Pito) are so impressed with my improvement over the past six months that they are now talking about "curative" and not just "palliative" treatments. They want to look at the longer, more focused proton treatment because they want *minimal cardiac damage* for at least a ten-to-twelve-year trajectory. That is very different from the original vague references to eighteen-to-twenty-month survival rates. The allopathic doctors, of course, attribute most of the healing to the chemotherapy, and I do think the chemo has played a very big role. I also think that the *alternative* healing approaches (including meditation and prayer) and the amazing and varied forms of support I have received from all of you have had a powerful synergetic effect. I do not think chemo alone would have produced this outcome. Thank you for that support!

The question is whether our insurance (Medicare) and United Health Care will cover the cost in my case. United will do whatever Medicare decides. This is a newer procedure with a less extensive database on outcomes, so insurance companies sometimes define it as "experimental," especially if it is not followed by surgery. (The first to use this technology, M. D. Anderson Cancer Center in Dallas, only has ten years of data, and while the data are promising, they are not as extensive as the medical or insurance community usually likes to see. Mayo has been using this procedure for a bit more than two years.) So I may be at the mercy of a Medicare official on whether or not we can take this route. That decision will be made in the next week or ten days. The daily trip to Rochester seems a bit onerous (ninety minutes each way), but the payoffs may be worthwhile. The backup radiology option has a well-focused high dose that hits the tumor, while about a 20-percent strength dose of the radiation hits a larger area, likely touching upon part of the heart and stomach. If that is the only choice, the two positives are that it has a high success indicator, and it could be done at Abbott Hospital in Minneapolis. The radiation itself takes at most fifteen minutes, and it would involve only twenty minutes of travel time. All of my Mayo doctors think some form of radiation is essential to turning this from palliative into a curative scenario, and my naturopathic doctor seems to agree.

Interestingly, the radiology staff I talked to was pleased that I was also seeing a naturopathy person and thought both the nutrition and hyperthermal therapy sounded like excellent decisions, offering synergetic effects with the radiation. So both the allopathy and naturopathy doctors are on the same page, which is not always the case.

* * * * * * *

My meaning-making reflection this week is on how cancer or another life-threatening disease can affect sense of time and one's narrative about past, present, and future. One thing that happens when in the midst of chronic illness is some confusion or ambiguity develops regarding time. As Kathy Charmaz puts it,

> Existing from day to day occurs when a person plummets into continued crises that rip life apart. It reflects a loss of control… What next? A crisis ends. A treatment works. Existence changes if health and prospects improve. Living one day at a time fades as someone begins to believe that tomorrow will come… A future begins to arise on the time horizon. (Charmaz *Good Days and Bad Days: The Self in Chronic Illness and Time*, pp. 185, 190).

Illness forces one into a subjective notion of time with time markers that would previously have been foreign to the patient: good days and bad days, a rhythm of treatments such that time is measured by infusion or treatment dates, and long-term projections about the future become foggy and uncompliant to any type of planning.

> Chronically ill men and women divide their lives into periods of illness and non-illness, crises and

quiescence, flare-ups and remission, rigid regi-
mens, and convalescence. Illness underscores and
marks events and sets boundaries between events...
During immersion in illness, the chronology overtakes one. Illness shoots by like a train that has left
the passenger behind, running after the caboose.
(Charmaz, p. 198–199).

I am aware in all of this how deeply I am a product of my culture,
which says that I should "own" the future, should move into it with a
take-charge attitude, and should demonstrate agency by planning and
being directive. As I have reflected on this and on how deviant seriously
ill people are from this standard, I recall how intrigued I was when I
read my first book by an anthropologist—Clyde Kluckholn. He discussed this notion of time in Europe and North America and how
non-universal those notions are. He pointed out that we in the United
States think and talk about the future *before* us and *moving forward* into
the future. However, the ancient Greeks and Mesopotamians thought
of time quite differently: they believed that we face the past—after
all, we can see it vividly through our memories—and that the future
comes up behind us and overtakes us. If there is any agency at all, it is
that we go *back* into the future and can only see the present as it comes
into view. We certainly are not in charge of the future in this imagery
or time metaphor.

I must admit that as a planner and a very future-oriented person,
I do feel like this cancer diagnosis has spun me around so that the
future does seem like something coming at me unseen from behind.
What sort of Mack truck is barreling down on me, or what blue skies
and fragrant flowers are about to enter my present time? "Planning
the future" really does seem oxymoronic. This ancient Greek orientation to time not only makes the chronically ill deviant from standard
American culture but also can be rather disorienting. Drawing from
Charmaz, we might identify several orientations to the future that
evolve in this situation.

The Dreaded Future: "By residing in a dreaded
future, people can live in silent terror and wait—

for months, years, even decades—for that future they know will come… The people disengage from the present. The past fades… Not surprisingly, feeling trapped by an uncontrollable future also traps one in negative emotions: anger, self-pity, and depression" (Charmaz, *Good Days and Bad Days*, p. 250–251).

The Improved Future: "Hoping [for an improved future] means looking to the future for fuller self-realization. People who do so desire or expect their future selves to realize present potential and to fulfill goals." While this may be a more hopeful and upbeat outlook, it may also result in deep disappointment and depression if the illness continues to dominate one's remaining life. (Charmaz, *Good Days and Bad Days*, p. 251).

The Truncated Future: This posture recognizes that one's future is likely to be much shorter than one had previously expected and planned for. One may decide to live what life one has left to the fullest, but it does accept the prognosis. The danger, of course, is that the prognosis can become a "reverse placebo effect." One expects to only live a short time, and that can become a self-fulfilling prophecy if one's body and mind become resigned to a shortened future.

How does one develop a positive and constructive stance toward the future that is both healthy and realistic? Pardon my embedded sociological bent, but it seems to me that there are two levels at which one may define the future, and both are important for one's well-being. At the micro (everyday personal level of interaction and living), one's spirit is affected by claiming some expectations for the future. I need to claim a stake in the future as a positive statement about my life and about my progress. Judy and I love to travel, and we still have places on our "bucket list" that we have not experienced. Somehow it has seemed dicey to buy tickets to Scandinavia or Greece or other destinations when my "future" is uncertain. We are also considering another human rights delegation to Guatemala, but my treatments, energy levels, and ability to eat local foods seem unclear. We finally decided that *not* planning for the future is a clear lack of confidence in my healing or remission. In the previous chronicle entry, I noted that Nobel prize-winning molecular biologist Elizabeth Blackburn and psychologist Elissa Epel have written that "our cells are listening to our thoughts" (*The Telomere Effect: A Revolutionary Approach to Living Younger, Healthier, Longer*). This idea resonates with me as having some measure of substance, and I need to be less tentative about the future. With that in mind, Judy and I have booked a Road Scholar (it used to be called Elder Hostel) trip to Greece for October—four days in Athens and several days in Greek Islands like Crete, Santorini, and Patmos. Other forms of micro level future planning will be discussed below.

At another level, I do believe that a healthy person is a person-in-community and must be a contributing member to the larger social fabric. It is in that frame that Judy and I have continued to be active in both ISAIAH social justice rallies and legislative hearings as well as Global Justice Advocacy and Witness for Peace events. The Lakota, who have so recently been victimized by the Trump administration ruling to build oil pipelines through their water supplies in North Dakota, offer some wisdom on future orientation. The Lakota commend a standard—a timeline—for evaluating the ethics of a policy, or even a personal decision: *what will be the consequences for the next seven generations* (not just one's next quarterly corporate profits statement). If I am a person in community, then I need to look beyond my own personal future and consider the future of my grandchildren and their grandchildren, as the Lakota do. In other words, as a responsible human being, "the future" is not just my personal future but also the future of the community, the society, and the global social system of which I am a part. With this lens in mind, "planning the future" may not be an oxymoron after all. The issue is what kind of legacy do I (and we) want to leave?

Setting Priorities and Thinking about One's Legacy

Due to my diagnosis, I am more aware of the possible limits of my personal longevity, so setting priorities for my time remaining is more real—regardless of whether that "time remaining" is a matter of months or more than a decade. The concept of legacy seems real to me at this time. The *Merriam-Webster Dictionary* defines *legacy* several ways. The first is "a gift by one's will, especially of money or other personal property." I must admit that I find the tertiary meaning of legacy more compelling: "something transmitted by or received from an ancestor or predecessor or from the past." The key synonym for legacy is "a gift" especially to a future generation. Gifts, of course, can be of many types and forms.

Over the past two weeks, Judy and I have addressed the first meaning by "taking care of business," including our financial situation. We have made sure our legal documents are up-to-date, and we designated bequests for justice groups and some financial care for our next two generations of Robertses. The bequests are important to us in having a portion of our resources continue to support social justice and earth justice causes that build a more compassionate world. So our focus is both macro (systemic) and micro (family). (I'm a sociologist, what can I say? The micro-macro link is a core concept in sociology. Individuals are *always in community*, and we are not *fully* human if we are not so embedded.) The interesting reality is that by defining "the future" more broadly—both in terms of wider community and subsequent generations—one begins to feel a sense of hope. Hope, of course, is good for body and soul.

With this in mind, we have updated our legal documents:

- Last Will and Testament
- Power of Attorney
- Health Care Directive, which in Minnesota includes:
    - Medical Power of Attorney
    - Living Will

We decided that for both tax and other reasons, a revocable durable trust is the most responsible way to leave some sort of monetary legacy at the micro level. Our children are old enough that we do not have to consider guardianship, which is often difficult decision for younger parents, but if you are reading this and have dependent children, do give this some thought. Regardless of age or health states, one never knows what catastrophic "Mack truck" may be about to hit one from behind (to use the ancient Greek/Mesopotamian metaphor about the future). The process of thinking through these decisions at this point in our lives was interesting, life-affirming, and oddly comforting.

The tertiary meaning defining legacy is the most powerful and most important, I think. It consists of gifts of words, images of integrity and a meaningful life, and examples or a model of a life well lived. What kind of messages do I want to have resonance for the next couple of generations in my family? What kind of wisdom do I want to pass on (assuming I have some wisdom worth transmitting)? How can I communicate a worldview at the micro level that conveys a passion about our engagement and agency at the macro level, especially regarding being in a society committed to peace and systemic justice.

This essay is already getting long, however. I hope I have communicated some clarity about the need to redefine what "planning for the future" might mean when one's own (my own) personal future seems tentative. The Lakota standard of seven generations is instructive for thinking about personal as well as social decisions about "the future," and it illustrates the limits of our individualistic mainstream culture's imagination. We need a broader lens and deeper vision. I will leave a more compete discussion about communicating and *living* one's legacy until the next entry.

Peace and love,
Keith

13

Communicating and Living One's Legacy

May 30, 2017

Infusion day at the end of May is cloudy (*but with a chance of meatballs*—as Judi Barrett puts it). It is a good time to reflect on this mesh of meatballs in which I am immersed. I have now met over the past two weeks with surgeons, oncologists, and a radiology oncologist. (I have also begun acupuncture treatments for esophageal cancer.) The long and short of it is that my situation has been pretty remarkable. The oncology staff all agree that my "reconstruction project" has been uncommon. As two of them said on separate occasions, "We are in unchartered territory with you, Keith. We are starting to be more aggressive with curative approaches, but we are having to make calls as we go" (paraphrased). It is almost unheard of to see such remarkable response over just six months with only small remnants of lung tumors—and what is showing up on the CT scan *may* be scar tissue or dead and not active cancer per se. Likewise, the enlarged lymph nodes are now virtually invisible except for the one near the esophageal tumor, and even it is perhaps one-fifth of the original size.

There is no evidence of tumors or cancer in any other part of my body and nothing below the diaphragm (so the kidneys and pancreas are "clean"—well… as clean as any toxin-clearing organ can be). The surgeon examined my hernia and felt that while it will need attention, it is not a pressing issue and can be put off until late fall or addressed in early 2018. My chemo today is chemo-lite since the oncology staff felt that six months of the most caustic chemo—oxaliplatin—was enough and was causing too much neuropathy. I am still in the recliner for four hours, but I now receive Herceptin (for the HER2 marker) and two other chemo combinations that are maintenance doses. I will likely be on something different—chemicals that enhance the radiation—when the later treatment starts on June 19th. I will receive radiation five days a week for five and a half weeks; at that point, the possibility of surgery to remove the thickened portion of the esophagus will be considered. My weight last week tied my all-time low as an adult, but I have regained five pounds this week.

It turns out that Medicare does not pre-approve most medical procedures. Because I am not listed as being in "curative care," there is a high probability that Medicare would not cover proton radiation after the fact, so I will likely need to do proton radiation, the older procedure that is not as tightly focused. The dosage they will give me is the dosage usually for people on curative regimen rather than a palliative treatment, and it can be done in Minneapolis. While there is some chance of damage to the heart (that could result in eventual hardening of arteries), that would be at least ten and more likely fifteen years down the pike. Irrespective of the Medicare issue, my oncology team met and were pretty evenly split on whether the proton radiation was justified in my case anyway. It is a newer and less "proven" avenue of treatment. So all in all, I had a rather extraordinarily positive report. With malignancy, there are no guarantees, but we seem to be moving forward in a very positive way. Thank you, thank you for your remarkable support! The compassionate buoying up has been in many forms—notes of encouragement and reflections on these chronicles, daily lit candles, prayers, energy work, and offers to serve as a chemo-sabe, to name a few.

* * * * * * *

In a very real sense, this is part two of "Planning for the Future When 'Planning the Future' Feels Like an Oxymoron." In the previous essay, I noted the contrast in the way we in the United States think and talk about the future *before* us and how we are *moving forward* into the future compared to the ancient Greeks and Mesopotamians who thought of the past before us—clear as day in our memories—and the future behind us and unseen. I found—and I suspect that others with life-threatening diseases have experienced this as well—that a stage 4 cancer diagnosis spun me around, and I found myself, like an ancient Greek, facing the past and wondering what unseen future was coming at me from behind. This notion of the past coming from behind to surprise and overtake us does not give one much agency—much sense of being an agent in control of one's life and in preparation for the future. Yet many medical scholars insist that sense of agency is a critically important element in healing.

I also discussed in the previous essay two meanings of "legacy"— as financial gifts to organizations or to family members via legal documents and as the more important nonmaterial gifts one passes on to the next generation(s). In a curious way, focusing on one's legacy brings together past, present, and future, for it requires one to reflect on past and future to deliberate on what one should be doing in the present to convey any legacy to the next generation.

One factor that can give a person sense of agency and a future orientation, when one's own corporal future is in doubt, is to examine the legacy one wants to leave, and my focus here is on one's *nonmaterial* legacy—the words and wisdom, the core of integrity that one hopes to leave behind. This is a tall order and a bit daunting to think about.

In a sense, I am still a boy scout at heart in that the guiding rule in our troop's monthly camping trips was to always leave a campsite in better condition—and better supplied with firewood for the next campers—than one found it. We always did… and I have always tried to leave any physical or social environment in better condition than when I found it. Whether I have been successful or not is another question, but that was my ambition. That, I think, is a type of legacy-thinking for those of us with a potentially life-threatening disease. Moreover, it is a focus that brings together past, present, and future so one can see the connections and strategize on how to leave something meaningful. Whether or not I personally survive, my community will continue, and my actions now may help it to thrive and be healthier and more life-affirming for all members of the population.

Much of what I will eventually leave will be words—hopefully some of which contain some wisdom. I like to think I have had a legacy through my word-centric (or framed less flatteringly, verbose) profession. For me, being a college professor was such a deep calling; it truly was a vocation rather than a job. I like to think I played some lasting or influential role in the lives of, at least, some of my students. They did nickname me, and for most of my last decade, I was known on campus not as Dr. Roberts but as K-Rob. I liked to tell myself that this was a term of endearment and not a swear word, but what do I know? I like to think that my other work on my campus—helping the college through accreditation by developing a first-rate assessment program, designing an innovative set of options for post-tenure reviews of faculty members, and developing a sound structure to the sociology major— has had some lasting positive impact. However, one never really knows for sure whether such actions play out as intended. I also hope that I have left something of lasting value in the teaching sections of regional and national professional societies. In virtually any occupation, one can reflect back on a positive legacy if one fulfilled one's roles with humaneness, compassion, and sensitivity. Words of kindness, support, encouragement, and affirmation of worth are contributions each and every one of us may contribute to a kinder and gentler world. Knowing almost all of my readers personally, I rest assured that you have left a legacy. If you know others who have left such a legacy, let them know, for we all need encouragement.

Insofar as words are part of a legacy, my writing, perhaps including this set of reflections on the meaning of chronic, life-threatening illness, may have some positive impact. I suspect, however, that the words (and wisdom) I am able to leave those I love most deeply—family members—are the legacy that will matter most. It is with that in mind that I began writing—for members of my immediate family and my siblings—love letters for their birthdays.

For my two granddaughters who are only eighteen months and approaching three, the letters will be given to them on their sixteenth birthdays. Hopefully, I will be able to deliver those myself, but if not, they are, at least, composed and ready for that occasion. In each of the letters to grandchildren, I have expressed my deep love and my joy in experiencing the world though their eyes. I have also expressed my hopes and dreams for the kind of person I hope each of these young charmers will become.

In addition, I have written love letters to members of my nuclear family and to my daughter- and son-*in-love*, as my mother always called the in-laws. In these letters, I have tried to express deep appreciation for each person and what they have brought to our family and to my own life. These letters can also be an opportune time to restore any damaged relationships—to seek reconciliation (if needed) and perhaps to offer apologies or ask for forgiveness if a breach exists. In short, I do not want to die with things unsaid. This applies to my siblings as well. (Neither of my parents are living, or I would have done the same for them. My mother wrote letters to everyone in the family on their birthdays of *her* eighty-fourth year.) My letters to my siblings recalled our relationships from our childhood and related some appreciation, or even humorous events, from yesteryear. For example, I wrote my sister (and I repeat here with her permission):

> You used to tell me that when I was an infant and had a soft spot on my head, you would reach in with your finger and scramble my brains. Well, I have not been displeased with the way my brain has worked, and who knows how badly I might have functioned if you had not done the scrambling, so good for you!

There were also points of appreciation that I wrote to Joyce.

> As the youngest in our family—and with a fairly significant age gap between the two of you and me—I often saw you and Bruce more as models of adulthood than as playmates. Bruce was more like a second father figure in some ways, and I often modeled myself after him as much as I did after Dad. Mom was a towering figure in the family in many ways—such a strong, intelligent, thoughtful, analytical, and compassionate person. Still, as my big sister, I don't think you realized the extent to which I also had you on a pedestal as we were growing up, and even (perhaps especially) after you departed for college. I was convinced your judgments were impeccable;

you were much more of a reference group figure for me than you can have known. When it came to interacting with girls—my peers—you were a standard against which my female peers were measured. If some of them would say or do something that I could not imagine you saying or doing, that was a turnoff for me. In addition, because I lived with two such smart, thoughtful, and kind females, I looked for those qualities in girls to whom I was attracted. Most guys were intimidated by really smart girls, but I found it attractive. Indeed, I think I actually had an unfair advantage in courting Judy, who was the academic superstar of our class, for many guys were intimidated by her intelligence, while I found it deeply appealing! So thanks for any edge you might have given me in approaching, interacting with, and courting the love of my life.

I have admired the way both you and Mom asserted an expectation of respect and how you maintained contempt for and rejection of sexist attitudes—even as early as the 1950s. I would come home sometimes having heard sexist remarks about girls/women, and I sometimes repeated what I had heard. You were both so dismissive of these absurd comments that I realized they were bigoted nonsense. In locker rooms, men's dormitories, and other "male bastions," I was often the guy in the corner who never repeated gender-based insults or objectification of women, and sometimes (probably not often enough) I would directly challenge those comments. I became one of the male feminists in graduate school, for the messages of feminism rang true to me. Thank you for the role you had in that shaping of my character.

I also tried to relate some poignant stories about things that influenced me that I doubt my siblings perceived. For example, I wrote my brother something that I realized I had never told him (and that I share here with his permission).

> When we were all still living at home, I remember being angry with you a good bit of the time. You teased me rather unmercifully—especially around the dinner table but at other times too. It was probably a nuisance having a kid brother eight years younger often trying to tag along... I used to get my revenge for your teasing, however. I almost always was the first up in the morning, and for breakfast and dinners, I usually set the table for Mom. I always gave you the old, often unmatched, silverware—not the "newer" silver plate ware with the fancy R on the handle. I am sure you have been devastated and traumatized ever since for this slight. Well... maybe not.

> Things changed dramatically in our relationship when you went to college. I still recall that on the first trip home—I think it was for Thanksgiving—you took me out to a restaurant for a piece of pie and a shake. I was flabbergasted, since I didn't really think you liked me very much. But you wanted to be alone with me. Incredible! You asked lots of questions about my own life and what was transpiring. If you were 18, I must have been about 10. It may not have been on that occasion, but later you asked me for my opinion about something. I have no idea what it was, but you also have no idea what a boost it was to my self-esteem that my opinion was worth hearing. I often had trouble in the family getting any kind of hearing since I was so young, and here you were asking me about something. That was important to me. Older siblings shape the self-worth of younger ones in profound ways, and this is one way you enhanced my (fragile) self-esteem.

I closed with a special note of appreciation for his role in my life.

> There is one other huge way you have been a remarkable big brother. We are in different disciplines, but we are both academics. In my career, I have had so many accolades, including highly prestigious national awards in the teaching area. Now my discipline is much larger in numbers of scholars and, therefore, has far more awards than your fields—Christian Ed, church leadership, and continuing theological education. Still, it would be very easy for a brother—especially an older brother—to perhaps feel some jealousy over all the "flowers" that have been thrown my way. You have always been one of my biggest cheerleaders. Do you have any idea what a gift that has been—your utter unselfishness in celebrating my awards? It truly has been a gift, one that I appreciate deeply. It takes a big person to do that, and you have been my "big" in more ways than one.

> With much love and deep admiration,
> Keith

Lori Hope (in *Help Me to Live: 20 Things People with Cancer Want You to Know*) writes:

> An oncology social worker surveyed sixty of her peers asking them how they would want to die. Few feared physical suffering because the medical practice of palliative care has become so widespread... Much more troubling was the thought of leaving things unsaid. While terminally ill people have the opportunity to tie up loose ends and prepare to die, those who die suddenly can leave behind a bitter legacy of longing or regret. (p. 135).

Words to our family members, spoken or written, can heal relationships. Sometimes it is easier to write things than to say them.

My hope is that in sharing words that I can leave behind, I might have a constructive impact. This is an important kind of legacy—words that heal and contribute to the self-worth of those I value so deeply. Yet another form of nonmaterial legacy is hopefully leaving a model for children and grandchildren—a model of healthy engagement as a person-in-community and a person of integrity. In this regard, I think we are always modeling some sort of values with our lives, especially with younger children and teens. We are so often *unwitting mentors*—we do not even realize whom we are mentoring, as I have learned from the moving notes I have received from people whose lives I did not know I had influenced.

So this is what I mean by *living* the legacy. The way we conduct our lives and the choices we make with resources and time send a message. Creating a more compassionate and just society is bone-deep for me and a central component of my faith; I hope that is communicated to younger Robertses. During this six months of chemo treatment, Judy and I have continued to be present at legislative hearings, discussions with legislators, phone calls to the governor, and rallies to support the disfranchised and the marginalized (including people of color and immigrants to our country). In some cases, we have taken three-year-old Ramona with us, so she has witnessed our involvement and our commitment to justice and mercy. Little ones are always watching and absorbing values and outlooks on life like sponges absorb water. We hope our faith (which, again, is not about superficial "beliefs" but is manifested in how one lives and acts in everyday life) is communicated as real and vibrant in guiding our lives.

Many of you are familiar with the assassination last year of the Honduran human rights and earth justice activist, Berta Cáceres. She was a remarkable woman who led many people by example and who embodied a sense of the sacredness of water (which was being laid to waste by corporate interests that valued profits above persons). At Berta's funeral, her daughter delivered a eulogy that ended by her saying, "Berta didn't die," and with her three siblings rising in unison to join her, they all said, "She *multiplied*." They dedicated their lives to continuing her work for peace, justice, and a sustainable mother earth.

Wow. What a legacy! She lived the legacy. Few of us will ever be in a position to have really big contributions like Berta, but often it is the small actions, the humane gestures, the micro-symbols of meaning that matter and that communicate to a next generation. The little things—the caring every day and showing it—do matter in big ways.

By defining "the future" more broadly—in terms of wider community and subsequent generations—one begins to feel a sense of hope. Hope, of course, is good for body and soul. It helps keep us focused on the future. At least, in my case, this has kept me from looking only at the past and has sustained me as I work through this "restoration project" of reclaiming physical health and of sustaining some sort of spiritual health in the midst of cancer chaos. I think I see time (and the future, in particular) less now as being either before or behind me and more as part of a timeline I sit on. It would begin with me as a little twit of about three or four. Through memory and reflection, I am able to move forward to see particular periods more clearly all the way up to the future. While many things are now faded or cloudy in my memory, the future is especially foggy or out of focus. Still, I have found that by contemplating our possible legacy, I once again regain some sense of agency and can move toward the future. Not only have Judy and I booked a bucket list trip to Greece in the fall, but we also have started to make plans for a river cruise on the Mississippi River for next spring or early summer.

A nonmaterial legacy can be expressed in words, wisdom, and modeling, and while a life- imperiling illness can ignite this kind of reflection, any time is a good time to consider what gifts one may leave behind. What is your (hoped for) legacy? I'd be interested to hear.

Finally, I received an unusual number of appreciative responses to my entry on "Awkward!—What to Say (or Not Say) to Friends with a Life-threatening Disease" (Chronicle 10). If you found that helpful, you might be interested in a book that the Mayo Clinic Chaplaincy Department recommends: *Help Me to Live: 20 Things People with Cancer Want You to Know* by Lori Hope. While she makes many of the same recommendations that I have made, she offers far more advice to friends and caregivers and has more empirical evidence for her claims.

Peace and love,
Keith

14

Optimism or Hope? Some Dilemmas and Ironies

June 13, 2017

This, it appears, may be my last intravenous chemo infusion, at least for a while. I am at Mayo Clinic, but starting next Monday, I will be receiving daily radiation treatments for five and a half weeks at Abbott Northwest Hospital in Minneapolis. The focus now is on the tumor in my esophagus, which has not been as diminished by the current chemo regime as the lung tumors (that are either "gone" or nearly so). My chemo regimen starting next week will change to chemicals that specifically enhance the radiation. After July 27th, I will have a month off any chemo. I have had to choose between wearing a pack and pump five days a week (if you have ever tried to sleep with a pump beside you in the bed, you will know it is not a cozy, intimate, or drowsy partner) or swallowing a pill of strong chemicals into a stomach that is likely to already be nauseous from radiation. Great set of options they gave me! I will try the pills and switch if necessary. As the radiation takes effect, it may result in temporary tightening of the esophagus passage, putting me on an all-liquid diet for a week or two. Nausea is another possible side effect, and neither of those bodes well for keeping my weight up. At my low point—which I have hit several times—I have been down thirty pounds; as of right now, I have gained six of those back. The most pernicious side effect of proton radiation to mid-chest is possible collateral damage to the heart. While it would likely not take effect for ten to fifteen years, the probable consequence is hardening of the arteries (which often results in a form of dementia). Ignoring for the moment the fact that some folks may think I have always been demented, this is the one long-term concern. My naturopath doctor thinks he can minimize some of these effects, but if people want a focal point for prayers or sending energy, prophylactic protection for the heart and arteries may be what is most needed right now.

There are many things to be thankful for in my life. My life has been full in so many ways, and now to have the "reclamation project" regarding my body working so well is more than one can expect. However, this week, we celebrated a milestone that deserves mention. As of June 7, Judy and I have been married forty-eight years. If we include the period when we began dating in high school, we have been a "couple" for fifty-four and a half years. Gratitude seems an insufficient word for having such a sustained and sustaining relationship and such a long trail of shared memories (all the way back to third grade… yep, really!). Life is good… and Judy is extraordinary!

* * * * * * *

I have written previously in this chronicle about how important outlook is to healing, and I have embraced the importance of positive attitude. Since penning those thoughts, I have read a lot about other people's experiences with cancer. It seems to be true that attitude plays a role in healing, and the three most important elements are hope, gratitude, and sense of agency (personal control). I continue to think those do matter, but I have also been humbled as I have read people's stories and heard how destructive admonitions to "be positive" can be for some people who are coping with cancer. It has forced me to reconsider, at least, some subtle nuances regarding optimism, hope, and attitude. My meaning-making seems to be in need of some amendment, for like many things in life, there are ironies and dilemmas in healing that one may not initially see.

In her book, *Help Me to Live: 20 Things People with Cancer Want You to Know*, Lori Hope indicates that one of the messages she has gotten from cancer patients is "I need to feel hope, but telling me to think positively can make me feel worse." I certainly do not think this is true for everyone with cancer—it has not been so for me—but dictums to "stay positive" may carry different meanings for some people and result in *dis*couragement rather than *en*couragement. So for meaning-making, this time, I thought I would try to unpack what is helpful or not and why this might be so.

What is the danger or downside of urging someone to look on the bright side? After all, people who think positively are happier, and one might expect they would be more hopeful. Positive attitude and sense of agency are critical to health, but when one is in despair (many malignant-maligned people even become clinically depressed), positive upbeat sentiments may sound Pollyanna-ish and be deeply hurtful.

Here is the problem as articulated by Barbara Ehrenreich: "If you believe that your recovery depends on your attitude, you feel this terrible pressure, like "How can I be positive when I feel so miserable?" (*Bright-Sided*). Many cancer patients are in deep bone-throbbing pain, experience profound depression, are immobilized by stark fear, or are very angry (perhaps at God); telling them to be optimistic is like asking them to jump over the house. Ehrenreich reports in *Bright-Sided: How Positive Thinking is Undermining America* that when she was diagnosed with breast cancer, she was faced with constant exhortations to "just think positively." She felt like people were trying to transform this life-threatening disease into a rite of passage; she was given the same formula as people who lost their jobs due to downsizing of corporations as the economy headed south—just stay upbeat and optimistic! She experienced this admonishment to be positive as both cruel and false. She was being told that she was responsible for her own cancer because of negative thoughts or deep despair. She felt blamed for her own demise.

This can weigh on a patient like a second disease. This double whammy delivered to chronically ill people had never occurred to me before, but I now understand it. Moreover, Lori Hope points out that hiding anger or fear—in order to put off a face of optimism—can keep one from recognizing symptoms that need attention. Pollyanna-like positivity can morph into a form of denial. Francis Spufford notes that this sort of "chirpy, squeaky, bubble-gummy reading of the human situation" was called cruel optimism by Saint Francis (*Unapologetic*, p. 11).

Note most of all that when the causality of one's illness is attributed to one's own attitudes, that may well undermine genuine hope, which really *is* critical to survival.

Ah, so we need to make some distinctions here about what kind of "positivity" is helpful and what is not. What is the difference between *optimism*, for example, and *hope*? I had not previously been careful enough in my own thinking about some important distinctions.

The *Merriam-Webster Dictionary* defines *optimism* as "an inclination to put the most favorable construction upon actions and events; to anticipate the best possible outcome." The *Macmillan English Dictionary* describes *optimism* as "a tendency to expect that good things will probably happen." Hope is different in important ways. Vaclav Havel has written that "hope is not the conviction that something will turn out well but the certainty that something makes sense, regardless of how it turns out." So hope involves a construction of the *meaning* of a particular situation or circumstance.

Dr. Jerome Groopman addresses the distinction similarly:

> What is the difference between optimism, hope, and positive thinking? Optimism is very different from hope. An optimist says everything's going to turn out just fine. Hope is very different; it sees all the problems and all the issues you're facing and then it chooses what appears to be the best path based on the information. (Groopman, *The Anatomy of Hope*).

Groopman insists that hope acknowledges the obstacles and pitfalls along the path but provides the courage to confront the challenges and the circumstances and sustains us in our efforts to surmount them. Hope, he says, is rooted in *specific convictions and expectations*, and those convictions, in turn, can block pain by releasing endorphins and creating a physiological response similar to morphine.

People hope that their cancer will be cured or, at least, go into remission; that they will live long enough to see a child reach adulthood or to attend that child's wedding; that they will not have too much pain when they die; that their finances hold out so they do not die destitute; that their grandchildren can remember them when they are gone; that they can heal a breached relationship and be granted forgiveness before they die; that they will experience peace of mind; that a political or economic problem will soon be solved; and so forth. Note that the substance and target of hope in each case is rather specific. Late in his life, my father-in-law (he was in his nineties) hoped very much that he might live past January 1st of a specific year because the inheritance laws in Ohio (his state) would change on that date. If he died after that, less would be taken out of his estate in taxes, and more of his financial legacy would go to his four children and eleven grandchildren. Now that is a very *specific* hope that would never have occurred to me as an ambition for longevity, but it was very important to him. (He did live to see his hope realized.) I hope it gave him a morphine high!

Lori Hope points out another distinction between optimism and hope: positive thinking and optimism are both mental constructs and intellectual processes. Hope is more connected to the affective side of one's personhood; it is fundamentally a feeling (*Help Me to Live: 20 Things People with Cancer Want You to Know*, p. 81).

From what I am reading and reflecting then, one may conclude that a generalized "optimism"—a "chirpy, squeaky, bubble-gummy, blind optimism"—is not especially constructive or helpful to healing, but hope, with some specific foci, can be very important. Indeed, lack of some sort of hope—some meaning and anticipation—may well impair health (Ernest Rosenbaum, *Inner Fire: Your Will to Live*). When doctors, nurses, friends, and caregivers project a sense of hopelessness and express their fears, it can create the self-fulfilling prophecy that I have earlier called a "reverse placebo." If I do not expect to get better or I expect to die in eighteen months, the chances are good I will live up (down?) to that prediction. By contrast, Norman Cousins writes, "The capacity for hope is the most significant fact of life. It provides human beings with a sense of destination and the energy to get started" (*Anatomy of an Illness*). So how do we generate viable, sustaining hope rather than just optimism?

One avenue to hope is a sense of gratitude. Now gratitude is also a sentiment that does not come readily to people who are deeply afraid, angry, depressed, or in excruciating pain. Still, one can see deep gratitude in the writings of Walter Wagerin (*Letters from the Land of*

Cancer) even at those times when he is in severe piercing pain, and that gratitude pulled him toward hope. Margaret Carlisle Cupit (*Why God? Suffering through Cancer into Faith*) also points to the many times when she was in some brutal heart-wrenching pain, but a sense of gratitude bridged a gap for her to a more positive outlook. The gratitude took time to develop; it was not her initial default response. However, over time, this nineteen-year-old became increasingly aware of the support structures she had—the hundreds of people, many of whom she had never met, who were standing, acting, and in one case running for her. Especially poignant for her was a fundraising marathon for St. Jude's Hospital where she received treatment. She writes:

> I was in my wheelchair, and… we were lining the streets because the St Jude marathon was going on. It was rumored that this year, there were 6,500 runners. And we sat cheering and shouting and clapping because they were all running for us. And for one of the first times, I realized that I'm not the only one fighting my cancer. I've known that my family and friends have been behind me. But for the first time, the people who make St. Jude's possible, the people who donate to St. Jude, had faces. And they were all running past me. Strangers kept pointing at me and yelling, "This is for you!"
>
> I just wanted to press pause because things seemed a little bit perfect. I looked up and saw tears running down my face and the face of another patient's mom… I saw six girls from my school [nearby Rhoads College] run by wearing "Team Maggie May" t-shirts. I don't know how else to explain it but to say that I was filled with an overwhelming sense of joy and gratitude. (Margaret Carlisle Cupit and Edward Henderson, *Why, God? Suffering Through Cancer into Faith*, p. 94–95)

Not everyone will have such a vivid experience of the extensive network of support each cancer patient receives, but insofar as you can help the chronically ill in your love circle see that, it may foster gratitude, which in turn enhances a sense of hope and of positive energy. Just being surrounded by expressions of love and support may be the ticket to hopefulness, not exhortations.

Lori Hope concludes that "hope may lift the spirits of people who have received a cancer diagnosis. But it is the freedom to experience all our feelings without being judged, without having to hide our doubts, that makes hope possible" (p. 79). Let chronically ill people vent. Help them identify specific things for which they want to live and express confidence that these hopes are within reach. If the chronically ill person in your circle of love has a positive spirit and outlook, support that! I do think it contributes to health, and it certainly contributes to a higher quality of living. However, I, at least, will try to be cautious in the future about not chiding people who are not upbeat to be more positive since it may create a second layer of burden—a kind of blaming the victim. Instead, I will seek ways to foster hope.

Hope can sometimes be fostered with effective use of humor, so next time, we will examine—and perhaps be amused by—humor.

Peace and love,
Keith

15

Levity, Laughter, Humor (including Tumor Humor)

July 3, 2017

I am not receiving chemo infusions at this point. I get daily radiation for five and a half weeks (at Abbott Hospital here in Minneapolis), and that is supported with an oral chemo that I take twice a day. I do not have radiation today, as most Abbot offices and labs are closed for the holiday, so I will use today to write my chronicle updates.

As I reported in my last two chronicles, the tumors in my lungs had diminished either entirely or are about 15 to 20 percent of their previous size. Because the two remaining tumors look more like weird crooked fingers than a spherical tumor, the oncology team at Mayo speculated that what we are seeing may be just scar tissue, and that is why they decided to switch to curative approaches and begin radiation. As part of prep for radiation, I had both a CT scan and a PET scan, and the PET scan showed conclusively that there is no (measurable) cancer in my lungs or the main lymph nodes. The radiation oncologist said that the clinical speculations were confirmed, that the lungs appear to be entirely cancer-free. Therefore, the move to radiation was the right move.

I am not out of the woods. While the chemo I have been receiving for six months may have retarded any growth, the cancer is highly active in my esophagus. Hopefully, the radiation—combined with all the alternative medicine approaches I am continuing to employ—will complete my "restoration project." All in all, the report is incredibly positive.

Radiation is different than I had expected. Using the CT and PET scans, extensive data is entered into a computer to identify the exact placement of my esophageal tumor. After making a body mold to hold me in a precise position each time and marking me with magic markers, which the technicians use to line me up in the exact position using lasers, this enormous piece of equipment rotates around me so that radiation is always hitting the tumor but only hitting secondary organs for a few seconds. This reduces, but does not eliminate, collateral damage. The primary area for collateral damage is the heart, although cells in the heart regenerate more quickly than those in the lung or other organs. I will not likely have many side effects until the third or fourth week except for fatigue, which I *do* experience. I also have a lot of neuropathy, especially in my feet where it feels like my feet are both asleep—sometimes a challenge for keeping my balance. The last several weeks, I will be on a liquid-only diet, which I have already been forced to begin. My weight is down to what I was in junior high school—sometimes hitting as low as 150. (Ideal weight for someone of my height and age would be 176.) If the radiation works, it will all be worth it, and this Saturday, I will be halfway done with radiation. So let's think about more interesting things: the role of humor in healing—a more "fun" topic.

* * * * * * *

Norman Cousins (*Anatomy of an Illness*) struggled with an unidentified, crippling illness tentatively diagnosed as ankylosing spondylitis, but he recovered after "laughing himself into health" by watching *Candid Camera* reruns and classic Marx Brothers, the Three Stooges, and Charlie Chaplin films. I have tried to find belly laugh comedy that I could soak up, exploring a wide range of options. Much of the humor by stand-up comedians today is either so foul or so racist, sexist, and explicitly defiant of cultural norms of respect for others that I do not find it funny. I have watched Marx Brothers, the Three Stooges, Charlie Chaplin, Red Skelton, *The Dick Van Dyke Show*, *I Love Lucy*, Jerry Lewis, and many others, finding that I smile, but they do not result in the belly laughs I recall as a kid. I have even bought four books of *The New Yorker* cartoons but have only modest success with that humor. I do still find Smothers' Brothers and Seinfeld funny, but sense of humor is affected by geography, ethnicity, national identity, gender, historical setting, culture, level of education, "maturity" (as in geezerdom!), and other factors. *The Van Dyke Show* was hilarious to me in the '60s, but much of it is poking good-natured fun at the 1960s notions of family and marriage that are not so funny in our contemporary scene. Probably the best thing to get me really laughing is just the infectious laughter of babies on YouTube. These are examples: www.youtube.com/watch?v=ZAmZucyzyZM and www.youtube.com/watch?v=L49VXZwfup8. It is amusing to see what babies find incongruous or outrageous.

So Norman Cousins argued that laughter itself was healing, and I think he had a valid point. Something about laughter cheers the soul, even as it distracts one from painful or negative situations. As Proverbs (17:22) puts it, "A merry heart does good like medicine." Still, I do think something more profound is also going on with most humor as healing.

Among the definitions of *humor* in the *Merriam-Webster Dictionary* is this one: "the mental faculty of discovering, expressing, or appreciating the ludicrous or absurdly incongruous." In a similar vein, Elton Trueblood maintained that humor involves an ability to turn a conventional way of seeing things on its head. That is why a humorous line is witty or funny—because it is so unexpected and forces one to see the situation in a new light. This is actually consistent with the work on the sociology of humor, a field of investigation that finds people laughing most vigorously when a standard social construction of reality is upturned by a comment that presents a radical alternative construction. We are taken by surprise. Indeed, the key is that one is unexpectedly looking at a familiar scene from a new and unexpected perspective; the heart of it is perspective-taking, an essential human skill.

Even the slapstick humor of classic comedians, like the Marx Brothers and the Three Stooges, often involves skits that have the characters doing widely inappropriate behaviors—like Charlie Chaplin tipping his hat to every woman whom he passes by and then also tipping it to a horse, or one of the Stooges who was asked to stir the soup and in absence of any other utensil used his shoe. Humor often turns "normality" on its head, and often normality does need to be upset, and our assumed meanings of conventional behavior need to be so overturned that our outlook is disrupted. Several of Charlie Chaplin's early films, such as *Modern Times*, are provocative critiques of aspects of modernization.

An example of a narrative that surprises is a story that one of my graduate school professors (Professor Jordan at Boston University) told a story to illustrate the difference between compassionate responses to suffering and structural or justice-oriented ones. I have used this story many times myself, and it often gets a laugh, along with thoughtful nods.

> There was a highpoint on a nearby mountain where people liked to go to watch beautiful sunsets, but the road up to the summit involved switch-backs and sharp turns along a cliff-side. One day a minor quake caused a mudslide that wiped out a section of the road, and the danger area was right around a very sharp corner. Many people went up the switch-back road and over the cliff to fall several hundred feet. Some died and many were very severely injured. Being compassionate people, the folks living in that region decided something had to be done, so being concerned, kindhearted [Christians? Americans?], they moved quickly... to build a hospital at the bottom of the cliff.

The story is obviously a metaphor, but it rings close enough to home—where we see programs for the poor, for the homeless, for ethnic or racial minorities that focus on ameliorative change (Band-Aids) rather than mutative change that corrects the structural problem. As a humorous metaphor, it *flips the meaning* of what we need to do in situations where a response is called for and change needed.

Trueblood writes, "Real humor, instead of being something light or superficial, depends on profundity. Kierkegaard concurred: 'A humorist rejoinder must always contain something profound'" (*The*

Humor of Christ, p. 22). Trueblood further asserts that humor and deep pain are often very companionable: "Far from laughter being incompatible with anguish, it is often the natural expression of deep pain" (p. 23). Moreover, humor typically involves clever exposition or highlighting of an unspoken contradiction, paradox, or irony; this explication is amusing when it is made explicit.

Still, the comedic element is the ingenuity in revealing something mundane from a novel perspective. In short, and consistent with the themes of these essays, humor involves twists and turns of *meaning* and often involves *meaning-making* in painful situations. This is meaning-making that can create laughter and levity and, thereby, can enhance healing. "To laugh," writes Trueblood, "is to see beyond the transitoriness of events and thus to be Jovelike—that is [to be] *jovial*" (p. 55).

While Trueblood seems to me to have overstated his case—much slapstick humor does not seem to me to have much depth or profundity—I do think he is correct that humor is at its best when it is more than lighthearted amusement; it can turn us to new ways of seeing things and transform a social setting or a social context into something different. Tensions can be eased, adversaries can laugh at themselves and see how foolish they must seem to outsiders or to the other, and the mood in a room or the spirit of a crowd may be lightened. Humor—if it truly has some depth—can shift the focus of a group or turn the mood around. The same is true for those dealing with chronic illness. Part of the reason it's effective is that laughter itself is rejuvenating, but it is also true that humor can spin one toward a different definition of the situation—a different meaning attributed to the circumstances one faces.

Humor often is a tool of oppressed or subjugated minority groups trying to redefine reality and, thereby, make the norms of the oppressive group seem ludicrous. It should not be surprising that so very many comedians in the past fifty years are people of color, especially those from African American communities. When Dick Gregory would mock the three cognitively challenged cousins—Ku, Klux, and Klan—he would get strong laughter from his audience as he made these racists look ridiculous and laughable. This is redefining the meaning of how the group defines itself.

Likewise, Jews are greatly overrepresented among humorists. Consider these famous Jewish comedians, and these are only a beginning of any complete list: the Marx Brothers, the Three Stooges, George Burns, Jack Benny, Milton Berle, Sid Caesar, Carl Reiner, Neil Simon, Woody Allen, Mel Brooks, Henny Youngman, Jonathan Katz, Jackie Mason, Don Rickles, Buddy Hackett, Rodney Dangerfield, Lenny Bruce, Gilda Radner, Andy Kaufman, Jerry Seinfeld, Larry David, Adam Sandler, Ben Stiller, Sarah Silverman, Andy Samberg, Judd Apatow, and Jon Stewart. Indeed, Arie Sover, Professor of Communications and Humor Studies at Ashkelon Academic College in Israel, wrote his doctoral dissertation on humor, and he insists that in the late 1970s, 80 percent of comedians in the United States were Jewish. (Quoted by Ayelett Shanin "What Makes Jews So Funny?" www.haaretz.com/jewish/features/.premium-1.704093.)

So liberals and those experiencing subjugation have often used humor—the redefining of something acceptable and normal as preposterous, nonsensical, farcical—as a method to change society. This is part of the genius of Jon Stewart in *The Daily Show*. Conservatives over the years have responded using their own humor.

When liberals began to stress sensitivity to language usage—terms and epitaphs that made people feel stigmatized and unwelcome in a social setting or organization, including women who felt harassed by sexually explicit references to their bodies—conservatives made that look foolish. While still a student at Dartmouth College, Dinesh D'Souza responded by making sensitivity to language and "hospitality standards" seem both absurd and a violation of freedom of speech norms. He did so simply by coining a term that is still used widely— *politically correct.*

The phrase "politically correct" was originated as a humor term directed at progressives who were depicted as controlling people's speech and freedom of expression. It makes progressives who object to harassing or racist language seem ludicrous and ridiculous. Insofar as it has put liberals on the defensive, it has worked as intended. Unfortunately, some university administrators really have abused hospitality language standards and turned the situation into a *power play* rather than a *teachable moment*, as it should be. "Politically correct" is a term I *absolutely* refuse to use, but I recognize it as humor that redefined a specific behavior as preposterous and offensive, thereby undermining a progressive social policy. That, of course, was its intended outcome.

Much of this kind of humor is making fun of others. Humor is usually at its best when it is self-deprecating rather than other-deprecating. Often ethnic groups or faith communities can make fun of themselves, and there is no edge or animosity, whereas if someone outside the community tells the same joke, it may be seen as hostile to that community. At a meeting of the American Sociological Association a couple of decades ago, the president of the association pointed out that sociologists specialize in studying groups and that groups often have names: a gaggle of geese, a pride of lions, a murder of crows, a gam of whales. What do you suppose, he asked, we should call a group or a gathering of sociologists? He proceeded to offer his own suggestion: we should speak of a "quirk" of sociologists—since we are a pretty quirky group. He got a huge laugh. Self-deprecating humor is often well received and sometimes even endearing. Another example was the person with a learning disability—dyslexia—who poked fun at his and others' tendency to reverse letters in reading and in writing (i.e. spelling). He wrote—in an organizational-activist-call-to-action style—"Dyslexics of the world, *we must untie!*"

A final example of self-deprecating humor is a young woman—a friend of our son—who had surgery and for a while afterward had to wear an external bladder. Now this bladder was noisy, often making fart-like sounds. It was potentially highly embarrassing, but she managed to defuse the situation by personification—giving her bag a name and a personality. She called it Steve, and she would talk about her "companion" lacking social graces. She was quick-witted and would have people laughing at Steve and his antics, talking either *to* or *about* Steve. By redefining her circumstance, she gave it new meaning; a terribly awkward situation became an opportunity for her to be quite charming and entertaining to those around her.

Tumor Humor

This preference for insider humor is often true with people who are seriously ill. Someone who is in the midst of a survival struggle with cancer or someone who has recently come out on the other side of the struggle intact can tell tumor humor stories. These jokes are more acceptable from an "insider" to the struggle than from a person who is entirely healthy, so that is worth keeping in mind.

In any case, a whole new category of humor has emerged in which chronically ill people make fun of themselves or their illness. Examples of this humor would include *I Barf, Therefore I Am* by Jerry Perisho or *Prostate Cancer Is (not) Funny* by Dan Laszlo. As Jerry Perish says in the opening paragraph of his book:

> We should treat cancer with extreme caution, but not with reverence, and we should not cower in fear. We need to rise up and knock the chip off cancer's shoulder. We should not be gently and respectfully handling it with kid gloves like it deserves the key to the city; we should be manhandling it with pick axes and blow torches.

Maybe, but perhaps more debilitating than violence in most enigmatic situations is to make it laughable.

Again, this humor in the face of chronic illness is best understood as meaning-making—it is an attempt to make the illness or the situation laughable, to deny it final power, to redefine—at least for the moment—what is happening. Here are some examples, the first two adapted from Robert Young (*How I Started Laughing: My First Cancer Joke*):

> I need a new wallet and go to a store and find a nice one, but it had a tag reading "Lifetime Guarantee." I turn to the clerk and ask, "Do you have anything that will at least last the rest of the year?"

* * * * * * *

A man elects to have a prostatectomy (removal of the prostate) and asks the surgeon to try to spare the nerves that produce an erection. Well, he goes into surgery and wakes up in the recovery room and sees his doctor.

Man: So how did it go?
Doctor: I've got good news and bad news.
Man: Give me the good news first.
Doctor: We were able to get rid of all of the cancer and to save the nerves.
Man: Wow, that's great news! What's the bad news?
Doctor: The nerves are there on the bed stand.

* * * * * * *

Doctor: I've got your test results and some bad news. You have stage 3 cancer, but there is more to it, I'm afraid. You also have a very advanced case of Alzheimer's disease.
Man: Wow! Thanks, Doc. Boy, am I lucky! I was afraid you were going to tell me I had cancer!

(With apologies: Sometimes tumor humor is less than sensitive to those with other diseases—such as Alzheimer's.)

* * * * * * *

Top Five Ways to Know You Are a Cancer Survivor

5.   When you use your Visa card more than your hospital parking pass.
4.   You're back in the family rotation to take out the garbage.
3.   When your dental floss runs out and you buy one thousand yards.
2.   You have a chance to buy additional life insurance, but you buy a new convertible instead.
1.   When you use your toothbrush to brush your teeth rather than to comb your hair.

* * * * * * *

A man hears from his doctor that he has cancer and only has six months to live. The patient wants to know, "Is there anything that can be done?" The doctor recommends that he first marry a medical technician who is well known in the community to be extremely narcissistic, demanding, and strident; then he and his bride should move to an isolated village in Alaska. The man asks, "Oh, dear! Well... will she cure my cancer?" "No," said the doctor, "but the six months will seem much longer!"

* * * * * * *

This one, also from Robert Young, is about death:

> Three buddies with cancer diagnoses were talking about death and dying. One asked, "When you're in your casket and friends and family are mourning you, what would you like to hear them say about you?"
>
> The first guy says, "I would like to hear them say that I was a great doctor of my time and a great family man."
>
> The second man says, "I would like to hear that I was a wonderful husband and schoolteacher who made a huge difference in our children of tomorrow."
>
> The last guy says, "I would like to hear them say, 'Hey, look! He's moving!'"

My dear friend, the fine sociologist Carla Howery, was a master at humor. Her sense of humor remained sharp always, and she could have people laughing at times when one would not expect humor to be found. I suspect that it cheered her soul. I do know without a doubt she lifted the spirits of her friends. Laughter may be healing and health-producing in itself, but true humor is more. It is the wit and wisdom to redefine reality and to make new meaning out of an ugly situation. May we all have the grace to do so.

I thought I might end this chronicle with some additional examples of tumor humor—this time in the form of cartoons. Enjoy.

Tumor Humor: Reducing Stress

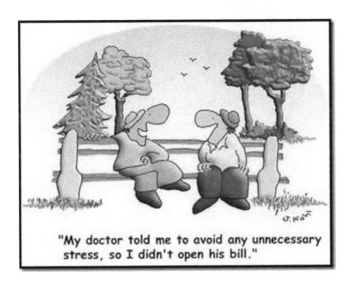

Post Brain Surgery Tumor Humor

Recovery   Botching the Job

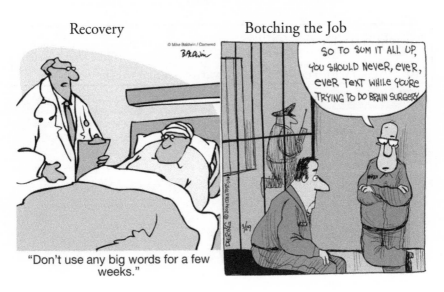

Physician Sensitivity and "Bedside" Manner

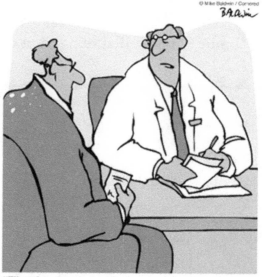

"The brain tumor's incurable, but let me give you something for that dandruff."

Peace and love... and laughter,
Keith

Sent to me in response to this essay:

https://www.wimp.com/hilarious-british-animal-voiceovers/

16

Hope and Healing: Omnipotence? Really?

July 18, 2017

Family, friends,

There is not much new to report on my health. I have completed twenty-one of twenty-eight radiation treatments, wrapping the radiation stage up on July 27th. The doctors are a bit alarmed in that I have lost nearly 20 percent of original body weight, dropping thirty-four pounds since all of this started. I now weigh what I did in eighth grade! Still, I have not had the most severe side effects of radiation, which include extreme nausea. I have also not had the usual "sunburn" from radiation. Perhaps I have just been lucky; it is also true that I meditate on the radiation table each time I received a treatment, imagining the individual cells of my heart, lungs, arteries, skin, etc. being wrapped in some form of protective Teflon and with radiation passing though without collateral damage to other organs. Many of my family and friends will nod "knowingly"—convinced that this was exactly what I needed to do. Others of you will now know for sure that I have clearly become a nutcase. The answer, of course, is *yes*. You are probably both right.

Regardless of the above, I do have some very exciting news. It looks like I have a publisher for these Kancer chronicles, and I am pleased to say it is a very solid publishing house. I sent off a four-page proposal just before noon and just before leaving for an oncology appointment at Mayo. The press's website said to allow *at least* two months for the editorial board to be able to have a response to any proposal. I had written to the managing editor. I got a response within three hours from Mr. Braden saying he was *very* interested. In fact, he said he was considering expediting this proposal. Maybe he wants to move quickly because I have stage 4 cancer, and he thinks he better get things rolling fast! In any case, he seemed pretty excited about the proposal and the four chapters I had sent him. We'll see how it goes.

* * * * * * *

My meaning-making essay this week has the potential to alienate some folks, but I hope you will stick with me to the end to understand how conventional understandings of God are often deeply alienating, hurtful, and hope-sabotaging for many people who are chronically ill or have really serious pain in their lives. It is an issue I have danced around and alluded to in several earlier essays, but it is time to address this directly. Many people—both members of faith communities and atheists—will view some of my assertions as shocking and as a departure from standard Christian understandings. This is clearly not the case, as we will see.

We have seen in earlier essays, especially #2 and #14, that healing is enhanced with reasons to hope and with a sense of agency (power to act). Agency is important because it strengthens the all-important feeling of efficacy—that one has the ability to affect change, to bring about some improvement in a situation, or to bring about an intended outcome. It would seem to many people of faith that God's omnipotence (all-powerful nature) is a source of hope and of efficacy. I am submitting here that more often it does the *opposite*. In essay #3, I wrote that the platitudes,

> *everything happens for a reason* and *this is all part of God's plan* are deeply offensive—even blasphemous. That would be a very mean-spirited God, indeed. Not everything happens for a reason; life sometimes has randomness to it, and that means accidents and illnesses simply occur. While these events are not meaningful in themselves, meaning

can be found and explored in any situation or circumstance, including realigning life priorities in a way that may be quite positive. Our task is to muddle through the circumstances we are experiencing, the conflicting information about treatments and strategies, and move forward with *agency* and *positive energy.*

Some people's faith seems so fragile that it will not entertain even for moment a different idea about God's power. This discussion may create some dissonance for people, but what I am asking is that readers consider how mean-spirited it is for many of us with life-altering—perhaps terminal—illnesses to be told that God is all-powerful and can fix the situation if God chooses. Yet God does not solve the problem or "fix" it. This is why affirmations of God's omnipotence often creates alienation and distancing from God and from a faith community at precisely the time when ailing people need that support. Why might this be the case?

Many theologians assert that God's supposed omnipotence is not only irrational but that it is disheartening and hurtful to those experiencing extreme suffering (see for example Edgar Sheffiield Brightman, *Philosophy of Religion*; Rufus Burrow Jr., *God and Human Dignity*; John Cobb, *Jesus' Abba*; Harold S. Kushner, *When Bad Things Happen to Good People*). The idea of omnipotence is also the major stumbling block that prevents many academics and many scientists from being Christian or theistic (Cobb). The question of God not being omnipotent is discussed freely and openly in major seminaries, but most clergy are afraid to discuss it with their congregations. Even Martin Luther King, Jr.—who clearly rejected the idea that God is omnipotent—was very circumspect with his language. He talked about God's *sufficient power* or God's *unmatched power* (Rufus Burrow Jr., *God and Human Dignity: The Personalism, Theology, and Ethics of Martin Luther King, Jr.*).

Interestingly, the notion of God as *not* omnipotent can be *more productive of hope* than the odd notion that God is omnipotent. It is time that someone was willing to say this "out loud" to the general public. Actually, Harold S. Kushner in his classic 1981 book, *When Bad Things Happen to Good People*, did say this very clearly. Whether one uses Kushner or Edgar Brightman or Rufus Burrow, the logical argument is that there are three propositions commonly held but which are in unresolvable conflict. These propositions are:

1.   God is good.
2.   God is all-powerful (omnipotent).
3.   Bad things happen to good people.

If God is good and all-powerful, why does God allow the Holocaust, or ethnic cleansing in Bosnia, or massive deaths from tsunamis, or horrible painful death via cancer—especially of a small child? There are Herculean efforts to explain these things away, but none of them ultimately are logical or "work." How can one possibly think that God would take the life of a child in order to teach the parent a lesson? The reality is that in order to pretend that these three propositions are not in conflict—to affirm all three of these as if they are not mutually exclusive—one must undergo some horrific intellectual contortions. These contortions are not even close to being plausible or reasonable.

The brilliant personalist systematic theologian, Edgar Sheffield Brightman (*Philosophy of Religion*), insists that "the eternal will of God faces *given conditions which that will did not create*" (p. 313, my italics). He continues, "There seems to be evil in the universe so cruel, so irrational, and so unjust that it could not be the work of a good God" (p. 318). He adds that there is no evidence that any source of power is infinite. Finally, power in and of itself is not worthy of our praise or deep admiration: "There is nothing worthy of worship in power, as such; only the power of the good is adorable, and it is adorable because it is good" (p. 319). So he concludes that there is a "givenness" about life and about the universe that is part of the nature of reality and that even God cannot control and possibly did not create. God works within those confines. (Note: Edgar Brightman was Martin Luther King's mentor and advisor in his PhD program, but Brightman died in the 1953 before King finished his dissertation.)

I am sure this sounds like heresy, and even some sort of New Age thinking, to people who have not heard the claim, but the reality is that these ideas have been around a very long time, including back to New Testament times. Certainly, it was part of personalist theology since the 1870s and was adopted from personalism in the 1920s as part of Whitehead's and Hartshorne's "process theology." I recall vividly a family reunion in the mid to late 1950s that involved a debate with my grandfather-preacher and my four uncles—two with PhDs in theology and one with a master's degree in theology. (I was perhaps twelve years old). These family reunions often became miniconferences on theological issues, and that year, the question under debate was whether God was omnipotent. One uncle argued in favor of the idea of omnipotence, my grandfather mostly listened, but my uncle who was an extraordinary biblical scholar—Horace Weaver—argued compellingly against the idea of omnipotence. I was fascinated by the discussion since the notion that God might not be omnipotent had never occurred to me. My mother, her sister, and at least one of the other uncles agreed with Horace. My Methodist grandfather-clergyman, who was always open to new ideas, seemed transfixed by the discussion. I have never since then thought the idea that God might be limited in power was odd or remotely outside of the realm of Judeo-Christian thinking.

Some might respond that a god with no power is hardly worth noticing... but I did *not* say that God has no power. Neither the President of the United States nor the Chief Justice of the Supreme Court nor the governor of my state are omnipotent, but that is not to say they are *impotent* either. They have extensive access to power, but the power they have is circumscribed by other powers and forces and by historical factors. God, likewise, has "unmatched" but not "absolute" power. God is our champion, our support, our comforter, our sustainer, and is oh-so-loving, but God cannot just wave a wand and have the laws of nature suspended so I can be healed. I could never love, acknowledge, or worship a God that is omnipotent but is also capricious and mean. The latter is the only logical conclusion for a God that is all-powerful. I believe God brings healing power, but that healing power is not absolute. Sometimes it is not enough. I have no idea why it is sometimes insufficient, but it is true.

In any case, for me, the choice is not between a God who is omnipotent and one that is impotent, but it is between (a) a wholly loving God whose power is constrained and (a) thorough-going atheism. Let's put it this way, which parent would be more admirable and worthy of our honor and emulation: one who has spectacular access to power but is capacious and only occasionally uses it to solve problems her or his children encounter, or one who is 100 percent supportive of progeny and has some power, but that power is constrained by other realities? To me, the second parent is more admirable and more worthy of emulation and collaboration; the same is true of God.

Finally, I must say that as a scientist, the notion that God can just supersede laws of nature at any point and that randomness does not exist is so implausible that such a God has no reality for me. That is why the only reasonable alternative to understanding God as limited in power is to be an atheist. I do not find the latter intellectually or emotionally satisfying.

So far, this argument for a compassionate but limited God has hinged on logic or reason; it has been a philosophical argument. There are two other rather compelling issues that need discussion as well. One is the nature of God in human lives, and the other is the grounding of a less-than-absolutely-powerful God in biblical teachings—especially those of Jesus.

Most of us who are theists see God as relational. The word *relationship* is defined by *Merriam-Webster Dictionary* as "the state of being related or interrelated." This clearly implies some sort of interdependence. When we are in relationship, we are constantly changed by that relationship—our emotions can be affected, our attitudes may shift, and our outlooks on life may be modified. This is a core principle of personalism, the theology that Martin Luther King so ardently defended in his doctoral dissertation. The idea is that not only are we humans in constant process, growth, and evolution but that God is also affected by relationships with humans and by human history. This idea later became a central principle of process theology as well—God is always changing, always in process. Indeed, God has widely come to be understood as a cocreator with humans as history unfolds. God does not just determine the future; God and humans *together* shape the future. Collaboration—in this and all other instances—never involves one side having all the power.

One act of supreme love that every parent of teens and young adult children experiences is giving each child freedom to make choices—to live her or his own life. This was also a great gift of God to humanity—freedom (free will) to make choices. True love is never expressed with tight reins of control over adult children. However, sometimes freedom is abused by those offspring and is used to pursue self-interests at the expense of others or of the larger community. This is one key avenue by which evil enters the world and our own lives. God does not control all; once freedom is granted, it is not to then be taken away. Parents may be mentors to their children and may try to love them into a responsible life, and God does the same. In short, if humans do have freedom, God is not all-powerful. Humans have some agency. Archbishop Desmond Tutu summarizes this freedom crudely, perhaps, when he writes, "God would much rather that we went freely to hell than *compel* us to come to heaven." He continues by indicating how God gets things done: "God weeps until there are those who say, I do want to try to do something" (Dalai Lama and Desmond Tutu, *The Book of Joy*, p. 116).

What about the Bible and God's power? The imminent theologian, John Cobb, points out that this rejection of the omnipotent image of God goes all the way back to the New Testament. Jesus called God "Abba"—which translated from the original is "Daddy" or "Papa." It is an intimate form of address, as Jesus was explicitly rejecting the terminology of the empire: King, Master, Emperor, or even Lord. Jesus saw God as good and as loving and as an ever-present, doting companion. This is very different from the transcendent all-powerful one that many in the Hebrew tradition had previously adopted—God as a distant but powerful King. Cobb insists that the biblical record, if one uses the original Greek and Aramaic sources, depicts Jesus as worshipping a God that is not all-powerful. I cannot summarize here Cobb's evidence, spelled out in an entire book, but he is convinced that Jesus did not see God as a power broker (*Jesus' Abba*). My own uncle, the biblical scholar who influenced me at family reunions and elsewhere, insisted the same thing.

St. Augustine in the middle of the fifth century wrote, "We should work as if everything depended upon our efforts, and pray as if everything depended upon God" (*Just War Doctrine. The Catechism of the Catholic Church*, paragraph 2317). In other words, don't count on God being able to accomplish "the good" alone. M.L. King quoted this on several occasions and would add that God and human effort combined were virtually unstoppable. This position enhanced efficacy and sense of agency for the civil rights movement but with realism about limits of divine power. I am reminded of the story of two boys who dawdled on their way to school and while still half a block away heard the warning bell to get to their rooms. One boy dropped to his knees. The other called back, "What the heck are you doing?" The kneeler responded, "I'm praying that I will not be late." His friend yelled back, "Yeah, well, I'm going to run while I pray!" Can we agree that the runner had it right?

All of this seems like rather abstract theoretical issues regarding theology, so why would I talk about it here? The issue is that when someone with a major catastrophic or chronic disease asks why questions, people who assume God's omnipotence often put responsibility on God. ("It is part of the divine plan" or "God has something to teach you.") Such attribution of the cause of illness leaves vulnerable people feeling isolated, confused, and even angry with God. It serves no useful purpose and certainly is not comforting. Major illnesses are not a time to discuss the intricacies of philosophical theology, but one can be very careful about language. To questions of why, many and perhaps most of us who are hurting would rather hear this:

> Some things are random or are part of nature's laws and beyond God's reach, but God is on your team and is working with you to find some sort of healing. The healing may or may not involve complete cure. In fact, the healing may be primarily emotional or involve wholeness of spirit. While God did not cause this illness, God can help you work through it. The most important point is that God loves you deeply, unconditionally.

Now that would be far more comforting than to be given the message that God is in control of everything, but God may or may not decide to cure this illness. A God with constraints is a God that offers real hope.

I don't talk about theological issues with professional colleagues much (many of them are on this mailing list), and they may be surprised to hear much of this from me, but deep in my bones, I know that the great God of love and compassion is in my corner, is offering support and comfort, and is acting like a loving mother or father who wants the best and will do whatever to help the healing. Yet I also know that there is givenness to the universe and to life on this planet that even God cannot dismiss. Some things are random! Moreover, as a person with a chronic and potentially terminal illness, it is far more sustaining to me to know that a good but not all-powerful God is in my corner. I am thankful for that loving God rather than an omnipotent but mean spirited one who could, *but will not*, use power to solve suffering, injustice, and illness. So let all honor, love, and devotion be to this great, good, loving… and *finite*… God. Further, let us work with this God to cocreate a more humane society and world.

Peace and love,
Keith

17

Meaning Matters

August 15, 2017

Family, friends,

I have gone a bit longer between these essays this time. I completed the radiation regime about two weeks ago and expected to meet with my primary Mayo Clinic oncologist today (now postponed to September). Still, there have been some remarkable developments. When I was just a week from finishing my radiation, I was hospitalized because I could no longer take in any nutrition—even in the form of pureed soups. I just could not swallow anything but water. So I spend a night at Abbott Northwest Hospital in Minneapolis with an endoscopy the second day. Going in, there were several possible outcomes, the most draconian being a feeding tube directly into the stomach. The least intrusive would be stretching of the esophagus with a type of "balloon." The doctor determined that the latter would work, though I will have to have perhaps four more such stretchings or "dilations" in subsequent weeks. More importantly, the doctor was able to get a look at the tumor and also take a biopsy. He could see no tissue in the tumor that looked like it was still living, and the biopsy (which is only four samples, but still) showed *no cancer*!

The news was stunningly good. The doctors do not like to use terms like "cancer-free" when one has had stage 4 cancer since there may be microscopic cancer cells still in the body. So they opt for that awkward and somewhat threatening term, "in remission." This latter term communicates a good deal of ambiguity and lurking menace since the cancer may reassert itself at any time. The allopathic doctors also like to attribute full credit for the remission to chemotherapy and radiation. While I think these elements played a very critical positive role, I do think that the healing has involved a synergy of the many types of approaches I have employed, including prayer and meditation. Rather than saying the cancer is "in remission"—which gives the cancer agency and seems to put a crimp in hope for one's long-term future, I prefer to say that my body has experienced restoration and is now "in rejection" of unhealthy cells. This emphasizes agency of my own body rather than depicting the cancer as having agency and able to return at the time of its choosing. In any case, my body is now recovering from the treatments, and things are looking incredibly positive.

* * * * * * *

As perhaps the last of these essays for a while, I thought I could conclude with reflections on why meaning matters. In addition, I have been asked to reflect on what resources one uses—or at least, what resources I use—in making meaning in an ambiguous situation. Having cancer seems to me to qualify as an ambiguous situation in which one's previous sources of stable meaning are disrupted. Let me start with this latter issue.

As a social scientist, I am prone to seek wisdom and knowledge not from a single source; I look for triangulation. The idea is to use multiple sources of information, to resist allowing any one of those to entirely outshine or surpass the others, and to seek instead coherence in which all or most sources point to the same conclusion. In the sciences, something is considered more reliable if several different research methodologies have been used, and they all point to the same outcome. In the theology of John Wesley, the idea is to examine *Scripture, personal experience, reason* or logic, and *tradition* (i.e. the wisdom of the ages). The theology of personalism added *scientific insights* to this "quadrilateral," seeking to find the merging point where each of these sources offer complementary insights. I try to do something very much in this tradition.

The insights of my faith community are formative for me. However, those do not cancel or supersede reason (logic) or the findings of the empirical sciences. My own personal experiences both as a scholar and as a member of a family that affirms mystical, meditative experience has been formative. I seek coherence in ways that all of these sources of knowledge and wisdom can be complementary.

Sociology has profoundly affected the way I make meaning, and these essays are deeply infused with sociological lenses on reality. Although my career has been as a sociologist with deep commitments to scientific empiricism, I also am convinced that empiricism has blind spots. Empiricism tries to test what we know by systematic testing using the five senses. It has resulted in deep insights and profound changes in how we understand our world. I profoundly appreciate what science has given us in the way of knowledge. However, I also believe that there are dimensions of reality that the five senses may not touch; use of the five senses to construct knowledge is necessary but *not sufficient* for a holistic understanding of the human experience. To use a simplistic illustration, we know that arctic terns always know what direction is north. They have a strand of iron-like metal in their heads so that the magnetic forces of the poles always tug gently toward the Arctic and Antarctic poles. This magnetic pull is not one of the five senses we humans have, yet it is part of our world. I have studied First Nations enough to be convinced that—like some of our mystics in the Western world—they may be in tune with other dimensions of reality that empiricism misses. Whether we call these "spiritual realities" or "energy forces" matters less to me than that I am open to the possibilities of wisdom not rooted solely in the five senses.

Having taught courses on first nations for more than twenty years, I have developed deep respect for the wisdom and spiritual sensitivities of so many indigenous peoples in North America. However, few books have had as strong an impact as my recent reading of Robin Wall Kimmerer's *Braiding Sweetgrass: Indigenous Wisdom, Scientific Knowledge, and the Teachings of Plants*. Kimmerer has a PhD in biology with a specialty in botany, but after completing her doctorate, she returned to her Potawatomi people (related to the Ojibwa, sometimes erroneously misnamed by Anglos as "Chippewa") and was reminded that many elders who had far less formal education than she did knew far more and had more wisdom about plants, than she or than her university mentors. It is an interesting read. At one point, she discusses contrasts in English and Potawatomi language.

It seems that while many European languages insist on use of gendered terms, including pronouns that require one to specify sex of a person, Potawatomi does not do so. On the other hand, her native language distinguishes nouns and verbs as inanimate objects (nouns) or animate subjects (verbs). Moreover, there are not many noun forms but many verbs. She writes, and as you read this, think about how learning her own language became an exercise in making new and different meaning of lived experience.

> [In] the Ojibwa dictionary... all kinds of things seemed to be verbs: "to be a hill," "to be red," "to be a long sandy stretch of beach," "to be a bay." Ridiculous!" I ranted in my head. "There is no reason to make it so complicated... A bay is most definitely a person, place, or thing—a noun and not a verb."

> And then I swear I heard a zap of synapses firing... A bay is a noun only if it is *dead*. When a bay is a noun, it is defied by humans, trapped between its shores and contained by the word. But the verb *wiikwegamaa*—to be a bay—releases the water from bondage and lets it live. "To be a bay holds the wonder that, for this moment, the living water has decided to shelter itself between these shores... It could do otherwise—become a stream or an ocean or a waterfall, and there are verbs for that, too. To be a hill, to be a sandy beach, to be a Saturday, are all possible verbs in a world where everything is alive. Water, land, and even a day, the language a mirror for seeing the animacy of the world, the life that pulses through all things, through pines and nuthatches and mushrooms.

This is the language of animacy. Imagine seeing your grandmother standing at the stove in her apron and then saying of her, "Look, it is making soup. It has gray hair." We might snicker at such a mistake, but we also recoil from it. In English, we never refer to a member of our family, or indeed to any person, as it. That would be a profound act of disrespect. It robs a person of selfhood and kinship, reducing a person to a mere thing. So it is that in Potawatomi and most other indigenous languages, we use the same words to address the living world as we would use for our family. Because they *are* our family...

In English you are either a human or a thing... Doesn't this mean that speaking English, thinking in English, somehow gives us permission to disrespect nature? By denying everyone else the right to be [a subject]? Wouldn't things be different if nothing was an *it*?...Saying it makes a living land into "natural resources." If a maple is an *it*, we can take up the chain saw. If a maple is a *she*, we think twice.

(From *Braiding Sweetgrass* by Robin Wall Kimmerer (Minneapolis: Milkweed Editions, 2013), pp. 54-57. Copyright © 2013 by Robin Wall Kimmerer. Reprinted with permission from Milkweed Editions. milkweed.org)

I quote Kimmerer at some length not to debate whether she is right or what this approach means for an ecology ethic but to show how changing the meaning of something transforms how we relate to it. Meaning matters! It *really* matters! Changing the meaning of words for natural phenomena can transform how we relate to the natural world. I submit that the same is true for cancer or any other chronic and life-threatening disease.

Let me use another example that to me is even more poignant. A few years ago, Judy and I went on a Witness for Peace human rights delegation to Colombia (and led by our daughter, Elise). We met with people who had been tortured, whose family members had "disappeared," and who had watched family members gunned down by government agents because they dared to stand up for human rights or for earth justice. We were told an amazing story by Marie of the Women's Peace Route in Colombia while we were there:

> There were a group of 12 to14-year-old boys who had, under threat of death to their families, been forced to join one of the pro-government and pro-multinational corporation paramilitary groups. They were ordered to pursue and "eliminate" a group of indigenous women who had been exasperating the government and profit-driven corporations with their pro-human-rights and strong "mother earth" stances and actions. These were barely pubescent boys, but they were given powerful automatic rifles and orders to exterminate these women.
>
> The youngsters pursued the women resisters who eventually found themselves trapped at night on a narrow strip of land surrounded by water. The resisters found several canoes, but taking the canoes would mean floating downstream right by these highly armed adolescents. It was the only option. However, these were highly creative women. As they floated down the stream toward the encampment, they decided to sing lullabies to the youngsters. The boys were transfixed. None of them could unleash the barrage of bullets they had available in their arsenal. These women were no longer enemies; they were moms who were singing the same cradlesongs their own mothers had sung to them a few years earlier. The women floated safely downstream in their canoes and rejoined their families. The only thing that had changed was the *meaning* that was attributed to these women by the boys.

Indeed, *meaning matters!*

I have tried to illustrate this theme throughout these essays as I have tried to make meaning out of a struggle with cancer. I have suggested that "stage 4 cancer" is not a synonym for "terminal cancer," and I have indicated above that talking of cancer being "in remission" gives the cancer, rather than one's own body, agency in determining the future. I hope that I have been able to model meaning-making that is intellectually and theologically coherent and consistent.

In chapter 6, I quoted Viktor Frank, a psychologist and Holocaust survivor: "Never seek happiness in life or you will miss the mark. Happiness is not a goal to be pursued, but a side-product of something else. If you seek to engage in meaningful activity and lead a meaningful life, something far deeper than happiness will be with you—even if you are in the most hopeless of situations. Seek meaning, and happiness and hope and contentment arrive as byproducts." Making meaning via these essays is one way I have tried to stay focused on living meaningfully and constructively about my (and our) future. It has been enormously useful to me as part of the healing process, and I hope it has been thought-provoking for readers. I recommend to others who are dealing with a life-threatening chronic illness that seeking meaning and finding ways to reach out to others through and beyond the fog of illness is constructive. It is much more productive of positive energy than wallowing in the notion that this is the "battle of and for my life." Avoiding the violent or warlike "fighting" metaphors has been one of the better things I have done. I am convinced that how we define our lives—how we define the meaning of life events—matters in how we live. It may or may not lead to some form of healing, but regardless, it contributes to a richer quality of life.

Thank you to all of you who have been so very supportive during this struggle for reclamation of my healthy esophagus and lungs. Your concern and prayers have been received and experienced as healthy, positive energy that is healing.

Peace and love,
Keith

REFERENCES

Blackburn, Elizabeth and Elissa Epel. 2017. *The Telomere Effect: A Revolutionary Approach to Living Younger, Healthier, Longer.* New York: Grand Central Publishing.

Brandon, Mark 2005 "War and Constitutional Order" in *The Constitution in Wartime: Beyond Alarmism and Complacency. Durham, NC:* Duke University Press.

Brightman, Edgar Sheffiield *Philosophy of Religion*; 1940. Englewood Cliffs, NJ: Prentice-Hall.

Burrow Rufus Jr. 2006. *God and Human Dignity: The Personalism, Theology, and Ethics of Martin Luther King, Jr.* Notre Dame, IN: University of Notre Dame Press.

Cahill, Spencer and Robin Eggleston. 1994. "Managing Emotions in Public: The Case of Wheelchair Users" *Social Psychology Quarterly* (57:4): 300-312.

Charmaz, Kathy. 1991 *Good Days and Bad Days: The Self in Chronic Illness and Time.* New Brunswick, NJ: Rutgers University Press.

Clark, Candace "Sympathy, Biography, and Sympathy Margin" *American Journal of Sociology (93:2): 290-321.*

Cobb, John, 2015. *Jesus' Abba: The God Who Has Not Failed.* Minneapolis, MN: Augsburg Fortress Press.

Cousins, Norman 1979. *Anatomy of an Illness: As Perceived by the Patient.* New York: W.W. Norton & Company.

Cupit, Margaret Carlisle and Edward Henderson, 2015. *Why, God? Suffering Through Cancer into Faith.* Eugene, OR: Resource Publications.

Ehrenreich, Barbara. 2009 *Bright-Sided: How Positive Thinking is Undermining America.* New York: Metropolitan Books/Henry Holt & Company.

Giroux, Henry A. 2017. *America At War With Itself,* San Francisco, CA: City Lights.

Groopman, Jerome. 2005. *The Anatomy of Hope.* New York: Random House.

Hochschild, Arlie Russell 1983. *The Managed Heart: Commercialization of Human Feeling* Berkley: University of California Press.

Hope, Lori. *Help Me to Live: 20 Things People with Cancer Want You to Know.* 2011. Revised and Expanded Edition. Berkeley, CA: Celestial Arts.

Kimmerer, Robin Wall. 2015. *Braiding Sweetgrass: Indigenous Wisdom, Scientific Knowledge, and the Teachings of Plants,* Minneapolis, MN: Milkweed Editions.

King, Martin Luther, Jr. *Stride Toward Freedom: The Montgomery Story* 1958. Boston: Beacon Press.

Kushner Harold S. 1981. *When Bad Things Happen to Good People.* New York: Avon Books.

Lama, Dalai and Desmond Tutu, 2016. *The Book of Joy* New York: Avery/Penguin Random House.

Leach, Edwin. 1972 "Ritualization in Man in Relation to Conceptual and Social Development" pp. 333-337 in *Reader in Comparative Religion*. Edited by William A. Lessa and Evon Zartman Vogt. New York: Harper and Row

Quillin, Patrick. 2005. *Beating Cancer with Nutrition*. Carlsbad, CA.: Nutrition Times Press.

Reinhold Niebuhr, Reinhold. 1957 *Leaves from the Notebook of a Tamed Cynic*. San Francisco, CA: Harper and Row.

Remen Rachel Naomi, 2006 *Kitchen Table Wisdom: Stories that Heal*. New York: Berkley Publishing Group.

Servan-Schreiber, David. *Anticancer: A New Way of Life*. New York: Viking Press.

Spufford, Francis. 2013. *Unapologetic_Why, Despite Everything, Christianity Can Still Make Surprising Emotional Sense*. New York: HarperCollins.

Thurman, Howard. 1981. "For a Time of Sorrow" *Meditations of the Heart*. Boston: Beacon Press.

Trueblood, Elton. 1964. *The Humor of Christ*. New York: Harper and Row.

Stevens, Edward. 1974. *The Morals Game*. New York: Paulist Press.

Tillich, Paul. 1957 *Dynamics of Faith* New York: Harper and Row.

Wangerin, Walter Jr's *Letters from the Land of Cancer*. 2010. Grand Rapids, MI: Zondervan.

Young, Robert. 2000. *How I Started Laughing: My First Cancer Joke*. Phoenix5. www.phoenix5.org/humor/HumorRVYjok

APPENDIX

Questions for a Cancer Support Group

Chapter 1: Health Crisis—Positive Energies Needed

1. How did you cope with the original diagnosis? What emotions did you have to deal with and how did you get your feet back on the ground (if, indeed, you have done so!)?

2. In dealing with cancer or another major chronic illness, what is the role of support from family, friends, neighbors? Why does it matter?

3. How do you go about sorting out the various forms of treatment—modern allopathic, alternative approaches, "precision medicine" based on DNA testing, etc.—and which set of doctors or which medical center to entrust with your life or that of your loved one?

4. Who needs to be let known about this cancer diagnosis? Who will contact them and how?

5. What are the advantages of going public with this news, and what might be some benefits of keeping things more private? What are the drawbacks of each option?

6. How will you keep those who want to know updated? CaringBridge? Who will keep it current?

7. Despite the shock of the diagnosis, are there things to be thankful for?

8. How will you handle the flood of offers for support so you do have some support but are not overwhelmed? People close to you will want to reach out. What kinds of tasks can they do that would truly be helpful: transportation? childcare? cleaning? yardwork? grocery shopping? If you do not need or want help, how do you indicate that graciously so people do not feel closed out or rejected?

Chapter 2: Who Have I Not Told?

1. If you received a diagnosis of stage 4, how possible is it *not* to equate that with "terminal" cancer and to get a strong stance for facing this life challenge?

2. The author suggests that a prognosis (six months or eighteen months to live) may serve as a "reverse placebo" effect. A placebo is a harmless substance, medicine, or procedure that has a psychological benefit to the patient but has no real physiological effect. People sometimes get better even if the "pill" they have been given has no healing properties. It is a self-fulfilling prophecy that comes true because the patient believes it. The idea of a reverse placebo effect is that a negative prediction may come true because they believe the physician's prediction. It is also a self-fulfilling prophecy. Do you think this does happen? If so, how can we guard against it?

3. Are you willing and interested in exploring alternative forms of medicine or therapy such as acupressure/acupuncture, healing touch, Reiki, anticancer diets, hyperthermia therapy? Why or why not? How would you find these in your area?

4. Do you believe that agency—sense of being in control—fosters healing? If so, how can that be enhanced for you or your beloved cancer patient?

5. How do you respond to the idea that this is a good time to tell others how much they mean to you?

6. Why might it be important to tell people how much their life, love, and friendship have meant to you and to do so now?

Chapter 3: Allopathy and Alternative Approaches to Healing

1. In valuating various forms of medical treatment or therapy, the conventional approach is modern scientific medicine (often called *allopathy*, though the definition of allopathy is more complex than we need to explore here). This approach has very high standards of proof before a remedy is employed, often requiring clinical tests that control virtually all variables and are double-blind and crossover studies so that neither the subjects nor the scientist knows until after the study who was receiving which treatment; a crossover is a longitudinal study (usually, but not always, via controlled experiments) in which subjects receive a sequence of different treatments. The author argues that while this very high standard of knowledge is useful, it also limits knowledge when other types of empirical data—even though extensive—are dismissed as unreliable. Some things cannot be studied in double-blind crossovers. Do you agree with the author that the standard of "knowledge" in modern allopathy is sometimes too limited? Does it have "blind spots"? Why or why not? What does this mean about openness to *alternative* forms of therapy or treatment (acupuncture, healing touch, meditation and prayer, Tai Chi)?

2. Do you ever feel like you or your loved one with chronic illness is objectified rather than being seen as a subjective actor and thinker? What might be some consequences of too much objectification of patients?

3. Do you agree with the author that, though not proven empirically (scientifically), meditation, prayer, attitude and outlook, massage, and energy work (like Reiki) can have healing results? Why or why not?

4. The author suggests a Qigong meditation practice of expressing gratitude for parts of one's body and for one's many support communities may well have healing effects. What do you think? Are alternative approaches worth considering? What alternative therapies can you share with the group? What gives you confidence in this alternative treatment?

5. What processes or criteria have you found helpful in determining what strategies to use for healing (recognizing that not all *healing* results in *cure*)?
6. The focus on diet is that what we put in our bodies for nutrition can act like medicine or exacerbate the illness. Do you think diet is important? What dietary insights do you have for others in the group?
7. How might there be healing that is less than a full cure?

Chapter 4: Framing One's Reality and Plausibility Structures
1. The author suggests that to avoid cynicism and sustain commitment to a set of ideals or to hope for the future, we all need plausibility structures. These work, he says, at both the micro and macro levels of society. So *plausibility structures* "are social and symbolic systems that allow social constructions to seem plausible—even compelling—in spite of contrary evidence." Do you follow his reasoning? Do you think hope and cynicism can take over if we do not have processes that strengthen our worldview? Why do you think as you do on this?
2. Dr. Roberts insists that the most important plausibility structure is a community that has similar social constructions of reality and similar values. Why might a community be so important? Do you find you need a community? What serves as your sustaining community?
3. The author also discusses the mutually reinforcing myths, rituals, and symbols that remind us of and that sacralize (make sacred) our outlooks. What symbols, rituals, or stories help you maintain hope in the face of a scary cancer diagnosis and prognosis?
4. How might plausibility structures increase our sense of agency?
5. In his essay at the end of the chapter, "Sustaining Commitment to Teaching in a Cynical World," Dr. Roberts shows how symbols and rituals kept him energetic and committed to his college students. Have you had any similar situations where you needed support for your values and your

outlook on life? How do you avoid cynicism in the face of evidence that things are not going well? Share your experiences with the group.

Chapter 5: Why Me? Why Us? Micro and Macro Malignancies

1. Why does Dr. Roberts indicate that "Why me?" is not a useful question?

2. Do you agree that "Why me?" implies that the next person down the road might deserve this, but not me. Does the question itself suggest that good health is earned? Do you think that is true? Why or why not?

3. Dr. Roberts indicates that troubles at the micro (interpersonal) level may parallel ones at the macro (society, or even global) level. Is this true? Why do you think as you do? How might this affect a person's health when dealing with chronic illness?

4. Is engagement in large macro issues healing—since it gives one a sense of meaningful focus? What experiences lead you to your conclusion?

5. Dr. Roberts reports that in the 1950s, General Electric was trying to stress the power of individuals who had resilience and abiding determination. In their headquarters, GE hung a one-ton steel ball by a very long chain and then positioned a one- or two-ounce cork—to swing with a rhythm into the side of that steel ball. Within two weeks, that one-ton ball began to move, and within a month, it was swinging. Is this a meaningful metaphor for the kind of resilience we need in dealing with micro or macro calamity?

6. What questions might you ask other than "Why me?" Share with your group questions that you struggle with as you deal with malignancy or other life-threatening ailments.

Chapter 6: Faith, Values, and Healing

1. Dr. Roberts quotes Viktor Frankl as saying, "Never seek happiness in life or you will miss the mark. Happiness is not a goal to be pursued, but a side-product of something else. If you seek to engage in meaningful activity and lead a mean-

ingful life, something far deeper than happiness will be with you—even if you are in the most hopeless of situations. Seek meaning, and happiness and hope and contentment arrive as byproducts." How might seeking meaning be healing for you? What gives you meaning right now?

2. Dr. Roberts suggests that equating faith with belief is a trivialization of how deep and how pervasive *faith* really is. How do you respond to this idea?
3. Roberts remarks that "my healing focus at the micro level is that I refuse to be defined by cancer—to let that somehow take priority in how I live and how I relate to the world around me. I refuse to give it that much power over my life." How does one do that? How does one refuse to give cancer power when it seems to define much of our lives right now? Share ideas with your group.
4. This essay ends with Merrit Malloy's Mourner's Kaddish:

   > When I die give what's left of me away to children and old men that wait to die…
   >
   > Love doesn't die, people do. So, when all that's left of me is love, give me away.

   Does this speak to you? Why or why not? How might this express Malloy's sense of what he wants to leave as meaning for his life?

Chapter 7: Paradigms and Constructions of Reality

1. The author asserts that faith, like values, are those core convictions that shape how we live out our lives. Many ideas we hold in our heads (beliefs) are like velleities (things we *claim* to value but which are never embedded in our personalities, our actions, our daily lives). If faith is more about a life of integrity than it is about creeds and dogma, how might faith be important to your healing or that of your loved one?
2. The author argues that faith is "the lens through which one sees and makes sense of the world." How might your lens—

your faith—affect your health and your effort to experience or model some form of healing?

3. Dr. Roberts suggests that a paradigm, a cognitive framework or worldview shared by members of a group, has a profound effect on one's attitudes and outlook on life. He argues that a rational choice paradigm focuses too narrowly on self-interests and also lacks any sense of agency. Social constructionism maintains that humans are meaning-constructing beings and have agency. How might your outlook on life—the big paradigm that shapes your view of the world—influence your health?

4. What in this essay or other essays thus far in this book has resonated with you and made you think in new ways about health and meaning in life?

5. Dr. Roberts writes, "Whether I ultimately prevail over this cancer or not, I live in the meantime with hope and positive energy." Is he just completely naïve or does this make sense to you? Share your thoughts with your group. How might the ideas in this group shape your outlook and foster healing and healthy-mindedness?

Chapter 8: Living with Ambiguity

1. "One of the challenges for people with a chronic, life-threatening disease is *ambiguity*." Is this true for you?

2. How are you dealing with ambiguity? Are there ways you have learned to embrace ambiguity rather than have it create anxiety?

3. Walter Wangerin writes, "A serious disease invades more than the body's physical symptoms." Indeed, it is true. He continues, "It invades by creating an entire meteorology of disturbances… What it disturbs and tests is… the rest of me: my character, personality, faith, morality, virtue, the spirit's gifts as well as the spirit's vacuities." Keith Roberts adds that "the destructive meteorological vortex within has the potential to hurt those around me if my moods swing, I am unappreciative, or I allow the negativity within to leak out and infect others… How does one keep the inner storm and

ambiguity from disturbing those closest whom one loves?" How are you coping with the emotional roller coaster—the meteorological vortex within? Share with your group and listen carefully to how others deal with the emotions.

4. Roberts writes, "Am I a naive fool? Perhaps, but it seems to be a path that has integrity and potential for positive relationships and positive energy in facing this health challenge. It may be the best strategy to make sure the disease of my body does not seep into a disease of my spirit, a healthy spirit being essential to a healing body. Does Dr. Roberts's positive outlook inspire more positive energy within you, or does he just seem a naïve Pollyanna? Discuss this with your group.

Chapter 9: How Do I Name This Experience? Warlike and Non-warlike Metaphors

1. Martin Luther King, Jr. often cited a core principle regarding change: "The ends never justify the means, for the means are the end in process." He felt the means and ends must be congruent. Does this make sense as we think about healing?

2. Dr. Roberts suggests that warlike metaphors directed at one's own cells are less than helpful, and perhaps even destructive for healing. How do you respond to this idea?

3. How do you respond to the idea of cancer recovery being a reclamation project—rather like an environmental reclamation of polluted land or waterways? Does this imagery resonate with you? Why or why not?

4. What other kinds of nonviolent metaphors or phrases are especially helpful to you in thinking about healing from cancer? Does the idea or image of tending a garden and pulling out weeds work for you?

5. Brainstorm with your group images or metaphors for healing to see if the group can generate some new ideas.

Chapter 10: Awkward!—What to Say (or Not Say) to Friends with a Life-threatening Disease

1. Dr. Roberts writes that the comments to the effect that *"everything happens for a reason or this is all part of God's plan*

are deeply offensive—even blasphemous. that would be a very mean-spirited god, indeed. Not everything happens for a reason; life sometimes has randomness to it and that means accidents and illnesses simply occur." How do you respond to this? Has God had a hand in wanting you or your loved one to have cancer, or does it make more sense to say that it was random but that God can help us make the best of the situation and make it meaningful?

2. How do you respond to the following kinds of comments from people regarding your illness?
   - "God never gives you more than you can handle."
   - "You are going to be okay. I just know it."
   - "What's your prognosis?"
   - "Oh, my mom had it twice, and she beat it."

3. What other comments have been directed at you that seemed insensitive, or even offensive and hurtful? When and if this happens, what is the most constructive way to handle the awkward situation?

4. One "best friend" said to a young woman when she heard of the cancer diagnosis, "Better you than me!" How does one deal with such comment? How does one respond graciously?

5. If out of anger you respond harshly to a supposed supporter but later realize you may have isolated yourself and cut off possible support, how does one restore that relationship?

6. Do you find yourself not wanting to tell people of your diagnosis, or even hiding the illness, because you are treated as less of a person if seen as seriously ill? If so, what are the consequences of that decision?

7. Does sympathy—as opposed to support—make you feel less competent or less vital?

8. The author says emotional labor is work one has to do to make others comfortable with one's circumstances. What strategies have you found work well to put others at ease?

Chapter 11: The Challenge of Cancer to a Coherent and Healthy Self
1. How has this illness affected your sense of self or that of your loved one?
2. What ideas did you get from this reading on how to strengthen the ill person's sense of self, self-respect, and sense of agency?
3. If sense of self is largely shaped by what is reflected back to a person—in how others respond—how might you take that into account in interactions?
4. Charmaz says that "in crises, a radically changed present separates one from the past. Like a guillotine, the crisis severs the present from the past and shatters the future. Hence, ill people feel severed and swept away from their pasts into an uncontrollable present and future." What strategies might mitigate this sense of an uncontrollable present and future? Is there something friends and family can do that would be helpful to the chronically ill person?
5. If it is true that "our cells are listening to our thoughts," as Nobel prize-winning molecular biologist Elizabeth Blackburn says, how can we move toward less bitterness and less negativity in outlook?
6. How can we help people with chronic illness to use their own best self as a reference point rather than the "looking glass" of others?

Chapter 12: Planning for the Future When "Planning the Future" Feels like an Oxymoron
1. Charmaz seems to use a roller coaster as a metaphor for the emotional ride that a chronic illness can create. What metaphor works for you in talking about what you have been through?
2. If you are the ill person, have you had the experience of the author of feeling like this disease has spun you around so the past is before you and the future is behind you and overtaking you? If so, how does this affect you?
3. In thinking about the future, do Charmaz's notions of the "dreaded future," the "improved future," or the "truncated

future" resonate with you? How or why? Does some other image or description of the future come to mind?

4. Are you able to do some short-term planning of things that would be fun or deeply satisfying? If so, what are some ideas? If not, why not?

5. Dr. Roberts suggests that setting priorities and especially thinking about one's legacy can provide a sense of the future. What positive inheritance (not necessarily monetary) will remain after your death? Can you help your loved one identify positive impacts of his or her life?

6. The author identifies some legal documents that need to be in order before one's death. Have you taken care of this kind of business?

- Last Will and Testament
- Power of Attorney
- Health Care Directive, which may include:
  - Medical Power of Attorney
  - Living Will

Chapter 13: Communicating and Living One's Legacy

1. Roberts argues that one's greatest legacy for future generations may be the words and wisdom that an elder generation may pass along. Does some sort of writing—such as letters—seem to you like a workable way to do this?

2. If you are uncomfortable writing, would telling stories and speaking to future generations via videotaped recordings work?

3. What is the most important message you would want your children, grandchildren, and perhaps great-grandchildren (or if you have no children then your nephews and nieces or others in your life) to remember? Why is this so important to you?

4. Are there things you want to tell your siblings or other family members before you die? Are there stories or experiences that need to be shared? What might some of those be? Can you share them with your group?

5. Are there things you need to apologize for, ask for forgiveness, or seek reconciliation with important people in your life? How will you do that?

6. Are there ways in which your conduct of your life has been a message—a *living* of the legacy? What might those messages be?

7. Does focusing on legacy help you or your ill loved one get a renewed sense of the future? Why or why not?

Chapter 14: Optimism or Hope? Some Dilemmas and Ironies

1. Lori Hope writes that one of the messages she has gotten from cancer patients is "I need to feel hope, but telling me to think positively can make me feel worse." Has the message of thinking positively felt oppressive or like you were responsible for your own illness? Why or why not?

2. Does the message that optimism and hope are not the same and that it is hope that contributes to health seem to ring true in your experience? Explain.

3. What specifically do you hope for at this point in your life?

4. Cancer survivor Margaret Cupit describes (in *Why, God?*) watching a marathon fund-raiser for cancer patients and being filled with gratitude. Does her experience resonant with you? What gives you a deep sense of gratitude? How might gratitude be related to hope in your healing journey?

5. Lori Hope (in *Help Me to Live: 20 Things People with Cancer Want You to Know*) concludes that "hope may lift the spirits of people who have received a cancer diagnosis. But it is the freedom to experience all our feelings without being judged, without having to hide our doubts, that makes hope possible." If you are a caregiver or support person for a cancer patient, how might you—without judgment—facilitate expression of the full range of emotions that the cancer patient might feel?

Chapter 15: Levity, Laughter, Humor (including Tumor Humor)

1. How do you respond to the idea of laughing at cancer? Is this something you can do, or is your diagnosis still too raw?

2. In what ways do you find laughter helpful or therapeutic?

3. What sources have you discovered that allow you to laugh, even if it is just for distraction from the stresses of the illness?

4. The author writes, "A humorous line is witty or funny because it is so unexpected and forces one to see the situation in a new light... Humor can turn us to new ways of seeing things and transform a social setting or a social context into something different. Part of the reason it's effective is that humor can spin one toward a different definition of the situation—a different meaning attributed to the circumstances one faces." How might humor help you get different—perhaps less weighty—perspectives on your chronic illness?

5. Did you find any of the tumor humor Roberts shared in the essay lifted your spirits—even temporarily? Explain.

6. Share with the group some of your favorite jokes. Especially relevant might be jokes about the medical field.

Chapter 16: Hope and Healing: Omnipotence? Really?

1. Has this illness brought you closer to God and strengthened your faith or alienated you from God and your faith community? Why?

2. If God is all-powerful and also loving and this bad thing that happened to you is undeserved, does it leave you wondering why the all-powerful God does not "fix" it?

3. Some people find the idea that God is not omnipotent is deeply comforting. If there is a givenness to some aspects of nature and reality that God did not cause and does not control, then God is wholeheartedly on the side of the patient. Does this make sense to you? Is it comforting to think that God, like a loving parent, is doing everything God can do on your behalf?

4. If God is in relationship and like everyone in relationship is affected by relationship, then God is always changing and in process of becoming. Does this make sense to you? Why might this be a comforting idea for someone with chronic illness? Is God a dynamic God that is "in process"? Why

might this be a comforting idea for someone with chronic illness?

5. If part of God's 'limitation" in acting is because God gave us freedom, is this comforting? Why or why not?

6. St. Augustine wrote, "We should work as if everything depended upon our efforts and pray as if everything depended upon God." How do you respond to this?

7. Do you believe that most of us who are hurting would rather hear this: "Some things are random or are part of nature's laws and beyond God's reach, but God is on your team and is working with you to find some sort of healing. The healing may or may not involve complete cure. In fact, the healing may be emotional. While God did not cause this illness, God can help us work through it. The most important point to dwell on is that God loves you deeply."

Do you find this true for you?

Chapter 17: Meaning Matters

1. Does meaning matter when it comes to coping with cancer? Why or why not?

2. Jesus rejected many existing social constructions of reality in his day. For example, he rebuffed the existing religious leadership and valued priorities by saying that people were not made for the law but rather that the laws were made for people. Do you think Jesus would expect us to be bold in making meaning today, even if it means challenging existing norms and definitions of reality?

3. What resources do you have available to help you be innovative in meaning-making?

4. What is the most meaningful insight you have gained in these readings and these group discussions?

5. Have these readings and these discussions made you more hopeful regarding your health challenges? Why or why not?

6. What is the main source of meaning in your life now?

7. How might sharing your sense of meaning be helpful to others?

ABOUT THE AUTHOR

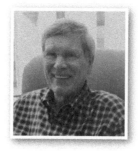

Keith A. Roberts is Emeritus Professor of Sociology at Hanover College and a nationally award-winning teacher. Theologically trained, his specialty is the sociology of religion.

CPSIA information can be obtained
at www.ICGtesting.com
Printed in the USA
BVHW07s1615070718
521037BV00001B/114/P